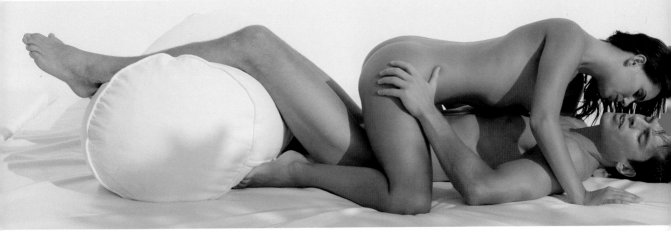

TRACEY COX
KAMA SUTRA

TRACEY COX
KAMA SUTRA

photography by john davis

DK

London, New York, Munich, Melbourne, Delhi

Design XAB
Editor Dawn Bates

Senior Art Editor Helen Spencer
Senior Editor Peter Jones
Production Editors Ben Marcus, Luca Frassinetti
Production Controller Elizabeth Cherry
DTP Designers Traci Salter, Marc Staples
US Editor Jane Perlmutter
Executive Managing Editor Adèle Hayward
Category Publisher Stephanie Jackson
Art Director Peter Luff

Illustrations by Gianelli (www.meiklejohn.co.uk)

First American edition, 2008

Published in the United States by
DK Publishing Inc.
375 Hudson Street
New York, NY 10014

08 09 10 11 10 9 8 7 6 5 4 3 2

TD282—January 2008

Published in Great Britain by Dorling Kindersley Limited.

A Cataloging-in-Publication record for this book is available from the
Library of Congress.

ISBN 978-0-7566-3354-7

DK books are available at special discounts when purchased in bulk
for sales promotions, premiums, fund-raising, or educational use. For
details, contact: DK Publishing Special Markets, 375 Hudson Street,
New York, New York 10014 or SpecialSales@dk.com.

Color reproduction by GRB, Italy
Printed and bound in Singapore by Tien Wah Press

It is assumed that couples reading this book are monogamous and
have been tested for sexually transmitted infections. Always practice
safe and responsible sex, and consult a doctor if you have a condition
that might preclude strenuous sexual activity. Challenging intercourse
positions might put a strain on your back or other body parts—do not
attempt them if you have injuries or ailments and consult your doctor
for advice beforehand if you are concerned. The author and publisher
do not accept any responsibility for any injury or ailment caused by
following any of the suggestions contained in this book. This is the
author's personal interpretation of ancient spiritual texts like the *Kama
Sutra* and is not intended to be an accurate representation of them.

Discover more at **www.dk.com**

contents

If there's one resounding message from spiritual sex, it's that couples need to put lots of effort into their sex lives. Sorry to shatter any illusions, but it's true: **people do split up when they're bored.**

introduction

I put my heart, soul (and other parts I won't mention) into writing this book—but I have to warn you, it's probably nothing like other books you might have read on spiritual sex. It's irreverent, not terribly spiritual in the "worship God" type of way, there's more than the odd "bugger" thrown in, and I've shamelessly mixed concepts, positions, and techniques from *all* of the infamous ancient texts. Rather than faithfully sticking to their original wording, I've reworked, reworded, and quite often taken some liberties with something some see as spiritually sacred. For this I offer complete and humble apologies.

But I did it for a reason.

The *Kama Sutra* is a wonderfully quirky, marvelously eccentric, slightly crazy tome, which happens to have **some absolute pearls of sexual wisdom mixed in among it all.**

There are many excellent books out there that *do r*emain loyal to the originals and the million-plus sales figures are testament to the fact that people are fascinated by its teachings. I've been decidedly sniffy about spiritual sex in the past, but I started researching it for my last book, *superhotsex*, and was suddenly seized with a need to bring it all to life again and put my own stamp on it. Because I still get the distinct impression most people think of the *Kama Sutra* as a book about sexual positions. It's not. It's a wonderfully quirky, marvelously eccentric, slightly crazy tome, which happens to have some absolute pearls of sexual wisdom mixed in among it all. Trouble is, if you do stick to the original wording, a lot of it doesn't seem applicable to modern life—which is why people have a tendency to skip the theory and instead ogle the pretty pictures of people with elastic limbs doing erotic acrobatics.

I figured if I rewrote the bits people often miss out on in a way most of us could relate to, you'd be far more likely to actually read them. And if I didn't pretend you had to take it all terribly seriously—because some of it is sooooooo out there, it's impossible not to laugh out loud—you might be even more intrigued. Then I added all the positions you clearly love on top of that, so you didn't feel cheated. And came up with something, I hope, that offers a fresh, innovative twist on the original. This book became a personal project—in more ways than one…

Being a huge fan of gloriously animal, throw-each-other-around-a-bit sex, the controlled element of spiritual sex put me off. But—and it's a big one—I graciously and unashamedly now admit defeat.

Rather than photograph it in the traditional way, paying homage to its Indian roots and going for a hippy-trippy environment, we decided to shoot it in ultra-modern locations. If I was going to do a modern-day version, let's set it in the modern day! Weirdly, though, some of the houses we wanted to shoot in, weren't so keen when they realized there would be (ohmigod!) *naked* people demonstrating (*what?!*) SEX positions inside it. Wimps. So I offered up my apartment as one of the locations. Wouldn't bother me. Why, I hardly noticed the gorgeous man, naked on *my* bed. Being the consummate professional, I calmly ventured out of my office to make cups of tea, without even bothering to glance at the couple cavorting on my couch. (Mainly because the models are ultra modest and put on robes between shots and you rarely get to see their bits once they're in position anyway. Dammit.) All went swimmingly well until one day, I popped out for a paper and, having the attention span of a two-year-old, managed to forget there was a shoot happening in my place in the three-minute walk from the store. So I merrily swung open my front door without having mentally prepared myself… to be treated to the sight of the male model, lying sprawled on my ottoman with everything exposed in all its glory. And what a glorious sight it was. So glorious in fact, I let out a rather *un*professional "Blimey!" which led to a lot of equally unprofessional laughter from the filming crew and the poor model looking horribly embarrassed (or pleased, still can't decide which). Oops.

Anyway, you'll notice the book has been structured in a certain way. The "top positions"— 23 of them—are original *Kama Sutra* staples (though I couldn't resist tweaking the names!). The others are inspired by various spiritual sources, including Tao and Tantra. Some of them look ridiculously easy, others impossibly difficult. But don't be fooled. A lot of what's actually happening can't be seen and the acrobatic positions aren't designed for traditional thrusting. All is not as it seems. As per usual, this book is for all types of people: straight, gay, bi, single, living together, married. It's for the sake of simplicity that I say "he" and "she."

Have fun!

Tracey X

erotic

exotic

exhilarating

exhibitionist

expert

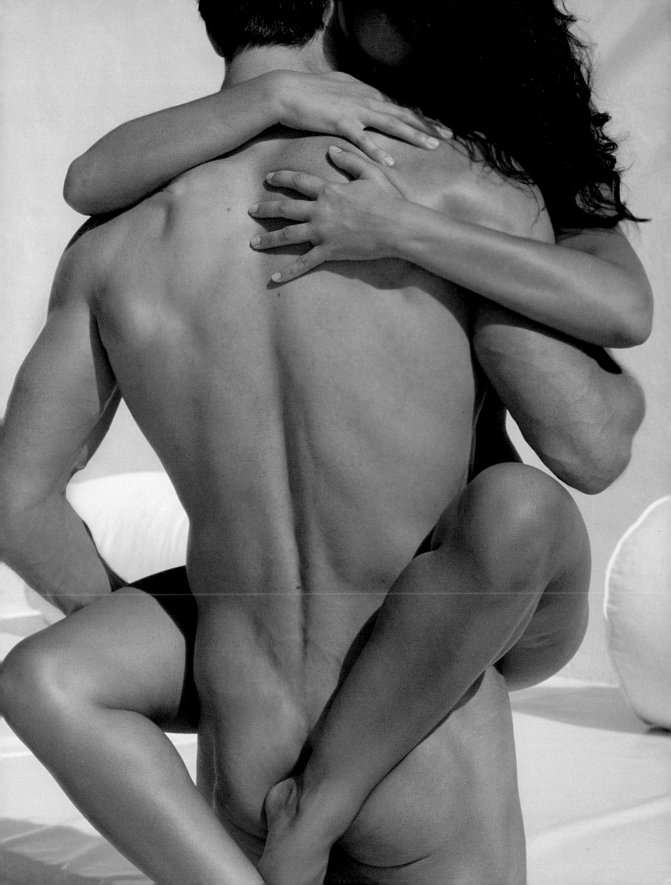

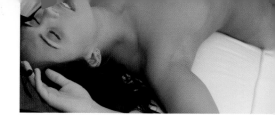

spiritual sex for dummies

WE TALK ABOUT TANTRIC SEX AND INFAMOUS BOOKS LIKE THE *KAMA SUTRA*, BUT HOW MANY OF US HAVE THE FOGGIEST IDEA OF WHAT THEY'RE *REALLY* ABOUT? HERE'S A CRASH COURSE IN THE BASICS OF SPIRITUAL SEX.

KAMA SUTRA

Like all things which keep us deliciously intrigued, no one can quite agree on the facts surrounding the *Kama Sutra*. We know it was compiled between the first and fourth century by an elderly Indian sage called Mallanaga Vatsyayana, but little is known of him. Some historians swear he was celibate; others say after studying ancient texts, he put the advice into practice and went for it! It's also thought Vatsyayana didn't actually write the *Kama Sutra*, even though he's generally referred to as the author. Folklore says he studied writings of holy men before him and discovered that Nandi, the white bull, stood guard for the mighty gods Shiva and Parvati outside their bedroom while they made love for 10,000 years. (And you thought that 48-hour romp was something worth boasting about!). Nandi swore never to speak of the sex secrets he saw and heard but, just like a fallible human, broke his vow and blabbed. The words he spoke "fell as flowers" and the flowers were gathered, strung onto thread, then woven into a book of 1,000 chapters. As time passed, the book got shortened and eventually condensed to 150 chapters. Vatsyayana managed to compact it into seven parts (only one of which deals exclusively with sex, by the way).

The *Kama Sutra* is basically a guide to life and love. It's addressed to men, but Vatsyayana heartily recommends young women also flick through it before marriage (with their fiancé's consent, of course!). At the time the *Kama Sutra* was written, there was no shame associated with sex—Hindus thought sex wasn't just natural and necessary, but sacred. A veritable sexfest apparently! (Time machine, anyone?). In 1883, the *Kama Sutra* was translated by Sir Richard Burton and Forster Fitzgerald Arbuthnot. So risqué was it for the Western world, they had to create their own company to publish it. Even then, it was only available through subscription and mainly read by scholars or upper class "gents'" with an appetite for erotica. Published for general release in the US and UK in 1962, it has remained the world's most famous sex book, even if most people are under the misconception that it's a "positions book" with lots of naughty drawings.

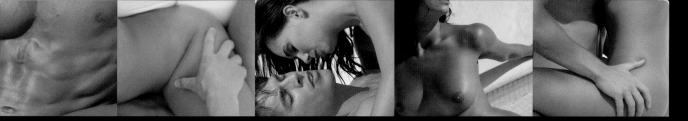

ANANGA RANGA AND THE PERFUMED GARDEN

Ananga Ranga, meaning "The Hindu Book of Love," was written in India during the 15th or 16th century by princely sage Kalyanamalla for the amusement of the son of the king. The attitude to sex had changed since *Kama Sutra* time—and not in a good way. Extra-marital sex was now severely discouraged (not that that's a bad thing!) and attitudes to sex had become rigid and inflexible. Shrewdly, Kalyanamalla envisaged most marriages becoming bland and boring, the more sex morphed into something to be ashamed of. He wrote *Ananga Ranga* to protect marriage from the sexual tedium he thought threatened it. Aimed at husbands who wanted to keep their wives happy, there's everything from fancy positions to kissing, scratching, spanking, and biting.

Written by Sheik Nefzawi in 16th-century Tunis, *The Perfumed Garden* was originally intended for men's eyes only, since Nefzawi believed bestowing pleasure was ultimately the man's job. Despite this, it's anything but sexist, dedicated to prolonging life-long passion. *The Perfumed Garden* stands out from the other books because of its writing style. The others inform, this entertains hugely with adjectives aplenty, enthusiasm bouncing from every page, and hearty humor.

TANTRA AND TAO

Tantra stemmed from a quiet but determined rebellion in ancient India, more than 5,000 years ago, against a male priesthood who thought desire and sex must be repressed if you wanted to reach enlightenment. The first Tantrics were teachers who thought sex was divine. So do the rest of us, though they meant it in the spiritual sense. Tantrics believe energy, called *kundalini*, flows through the body, running through energy centers or "chakras." Tantric sex opens up the chakras which helps move the energy to a point at the top of the head that produces pure ecstasy. The techniques are complex—it's serious stuff (which is why casual sex doesn't get attention).

The Taoists were a group of Chinese physicians who studied sex around 2,000 years ago. Their conclusion was that sex is necessary to provide physical, spiritual, and mental well-being. Hear, hear! Written before the other spiritual texts, Taoists, like Tantrics, believe energy is the source of all life. They also believe life is a balance of opposites and show how to balance the yin (female energy) and yang (masculine energy). Both forces are exchanged through sex—and it's at orgasm that they're most potent. Sounds like a damn good excuse to have more sex to me!

01

TOP POSITION

widely opened

A lift of her hips and a curve of her back means constant clitoral contact—and one very happy girlfriend!

How to do it

She arches her back and lifts her bottom, legs opened wide. He props himself up on his hands for support. Like all face-to-face positions, this one's derived from the missionary, except instead of having their bottoms planted on the bed, they're lifted high in the air. Not only is this a brilliant workout for her thighs and bottom (bonus!), it pushes the clitoris against the base of his penis providing friction during thrusting.

Why you'd want to

It's a perfect position for maintaining eye-to-eye contact, and great for watching each other orgasm. Holding her hips high gives him the feeling she desperately wants him inside her.

Hot hint

If her thighs or bottom start to ache, put some firm pillows under her (rather grateful) bottom and lower yourselves onto them.

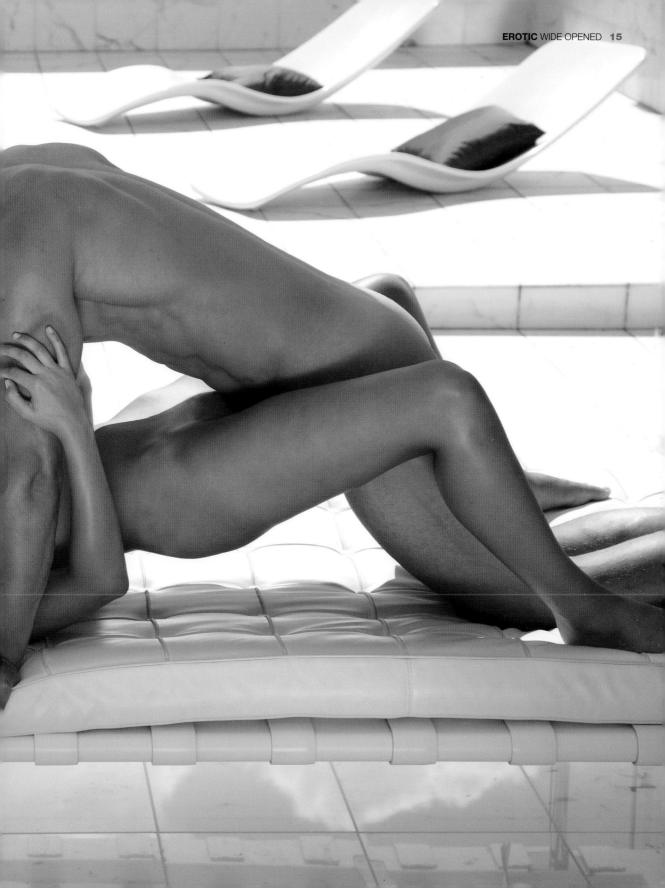

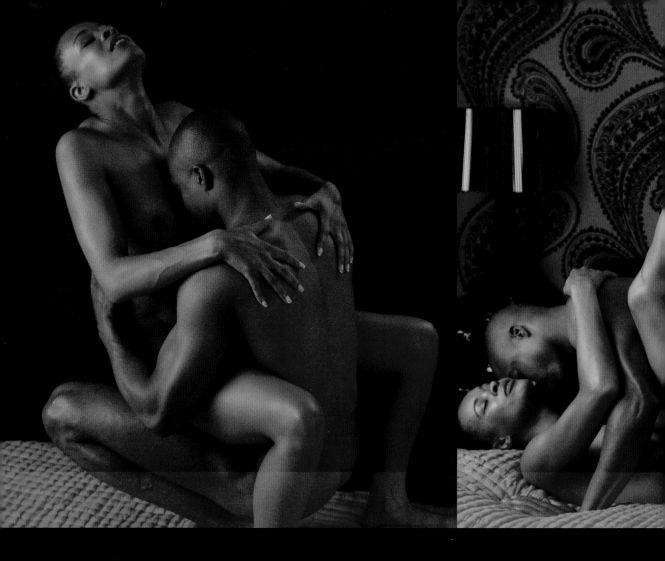

A twist on some old favorites

IT'S NATURAL TO MOVE FROM CHALLENGING POSITIONS TO COMFY FAVORITES LIKE THE MISSIONARY. USING THESE INNOVATIVE TWISTS KEEPS THINGS FRESH.

THE FROG

He squats with his legs apart and she climbs on board to sit on his lap, putting her legs over his. This puts his head—rather conveniently—smack bang in between her breasts (what luck!), the perfect position to nuzzle or lick. She holds his shoulders and keeps her feet flat on the bed for balance. He holds her around the hips. Rather than thrusting, he moves in a gentle rocking motion, while she squeezes her pelvic floor muscles. When his thigh muscles give out, he can roll backward and bounce her on his lap.

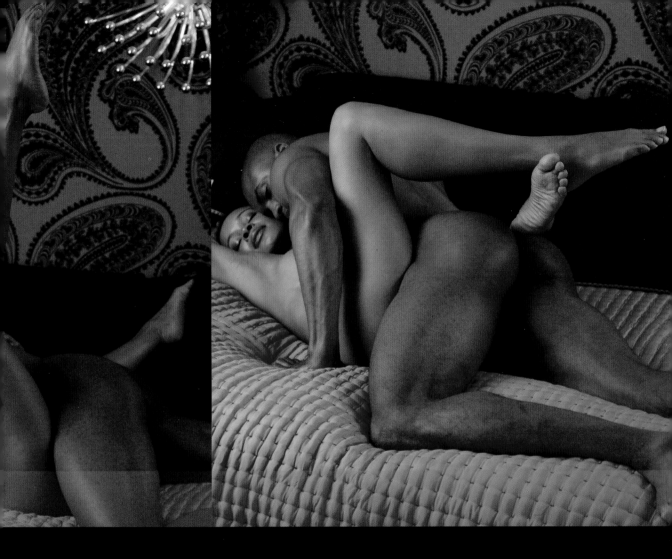

BALLERINA

She lies on her back and lifts her legs as
high as possible, while simultaneously
holding them as wide as possible. This
is called "yawning" in the *Kama Sutra*. Do
it for profound penetration and to get a
primitive buzz. It puts her in a vulnerable,
submissive pose, while he looks all
dominant and manly leaning over her in a
predatory fashion. It provides opportunities
for lots of lovely face-to-face contact for
kissing like teenagers and makes the
missionary position a tad more interesting

LOVE TRIANGLE

Move effortlessly from the elegant ballerina
position (see left) into a love triangle you'll
enjoy as she adjusts the position of her legs
to form a triangle shape. This allows him to
ride higher and penetrate more from the
side, altering the stimulation so neither of
you get desensitized. This pulls him deeper
into her and feels more intimate. Even a
slight reposition of the hips can make a
huge difference in how intercourse feels for
both of you, so alter your weight at regular
intervals to keep stimulation fresh.

02

TOP POSITION

rising

Her thighs being spread wide ups the eroticism, and being able to make intense eye contact adds intimacy to passion.

How to do it

She raises her legs in the air, making a wide "V" shape by holding her thighs open with her hands. He penetrates in the usual man-on-top position. Penetration is already pretty intense, but if she's feeling particularly raunchy and wants him even deeper, she should bend her knees and bring them up to her chest. Some interpretations of this pose include her putting her feet in front of him, pressing against the top of his chest.

Why you'd want to

This position shortens the vagina, making her feel tighter so it's a good choice if she has a large vagina and he has a small penis.

Hot hint

It's all in the angle of her legs—if he hits so deep it's more *owww* than *ahhh,* try legs together pressed on his chest and thighs squeezed, rather than parted.

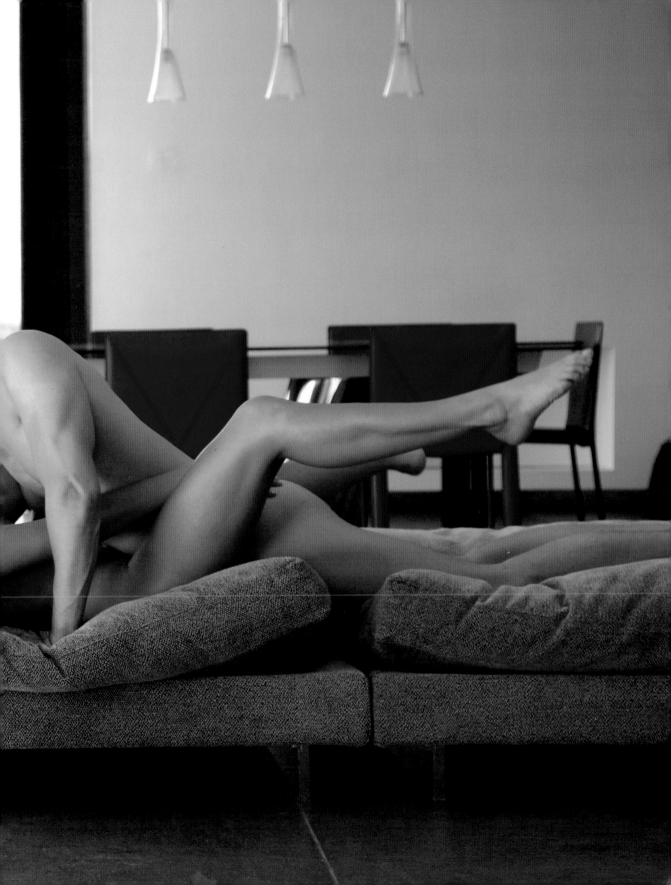

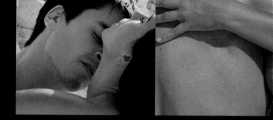

debonking the myth

SPIRITUAL SEX UP CLOSE AND PERSONAL. DOES TANTRA DESERVE THE HYPE? IS THE *KAMA SUTRA* A SACRED SEX MANUAL OR AN OUTDATED OLD TEXTBOOK? AN HONEST LOOK AT WHAT WORKS, WHAT DOESN'T—AND WHY.

As I've already mentioned, I was a late convert to spiritual sex. Being a rather impatient person (okay, drop the "rather"), reports of tediously long intercourse sessions had little appeal. Gazing into a lover's eyes for a minute or two might be sweet but, quite frankly, I'd be mentally bringing up which movie to watch after that. As for things like inhaling my partner's breath… well, that still makes a little bit of vomit rise in my throat.

Some take a look at the long, complicated pre-sex rituals and decide **takeaway is infinitely more practical than an 18-course banquet.** Especially when it's Monday night and their favorite TV show is on in an hour.

Being a huge fan of gloriously animal, throw-each-other-around-a-bit sex, the controlled element of spiritual sex also put me off. But—and it's a big one—I graciously and unashamedly now admit defeat! My initial assumption that spiritual sex was basically a lot of hippy-trippy garbage was wrong. Annoying, dippy, or dreary bits aside, there's some brilliant advice in those dusty old textbooks, most particularly in the *Kama Sutra*. (Which is a good thing really, since you've just bought a whole book based on it!) You need to alter your head a little because a lot of sex in the spiritual texts doesn't actually fit our definition of it. Intimacy exercises, like mirroring each other's breathing, are more romantic than lusty, for instance. But if you, like me, stay wide open (so to speak) to new ways of thinking, you might just become a convert, too! Before we get stuck in specifics, I thought a broad overview of what I think works and what doesn't, might be useful. That way we'll both know where we're coming from—and can get onto the business of coming.

WHAT WORKS

It puts soul back into sex Even though casual sex and one-night stands were as commonplace back then as they are now (Vatsyayana heartily encourages them—though there are rules to follow!), sex and intimacy didn't become separated from each other.

It promotes foreplay A basic rule of spiritual sex is to insist he waits until she is trembling with desire before even *thinking* about intercourse. Ironic that 2,000 years on, some men are still failing to absorb this simple message. There are lots of erotic kissing techniques and Vatsyayana also recognized female orgasm ahead of his time. Tantrics were among the first to acknowledge female ejaculation.

It isn't orgasm focused While orgasm is recognized as a type of nirvana, *Kama Sutra* sex is unhurried, with no pressure or official "finish." All the spiritual texts have a healthy disregard for the standard pattern of modern sex—four minutes from start to finish following the predictable pattern of kissing, fondling of breasts, hands below, (if you're lucky), a tongue, then straight on to intercourse and orgasm. Let's be honest: *anything* else is an improvement.

It keeps sex exciting If there's one resounding message from spiritual sex, it's that couples need to put lots of effort into their sex lives. They don't just allude to couples splitting up from sexual boredom, they point fingers at it. And sorry to shatter any illusions, but it's true! People do split up when they're bored. Put a tenth of the effort into your sex life suggested by the *Kama Sutra*, and it'll be one hundred times more effort than the average couple.

There's more than one way to thrust Traditional thrusting is great—but there's more than one way to have intercourse. He's encouraged to try lots of different thrusting techniques, choosing whatever best suits the mood. The end result is variety (joy!)— and often a rather pleasant pressure on the clitoris (even better!) There's no sex discrimination either: she's instructed on how to pump his penis, too.

WHAT DOESN'T

Ejaculation is discouraged Pure Tao teaches that loss of semen weakens a man and shortens his life, so ejaculation is permitted only when necessary. A quick phone call to all my friends got pretty much the same reaction: men were horrified at the thought of not being able to "let go," practically on their knees begging me not to advocate it; women were less concerned but most said they liked him ejaculating inside of them because it was both sexy and bonding. Tao also teaches men to separate orgasm from ejaculation. This certainly is possible— and I take my hat (and possibly top and panties) off to any man who's committed enough to do the training it takes to master this. I've just never actually met anyone who's achieved it. (Note to Sting: I am available for dinner if you'd like to be the first.)

Sexual rituals To say rituals are important to spiritual sex is a little like saying lots of people like vodka with tonic. If you're the type who likes a bit of pomp and ceremony, the complex (and sometimes seemingly quite pointless) preparations for a bit of in-out, in-out may appeal. Others take one look at the long, complicated pre-sex rituals and decide takeaway is infinitely more practical than an 18-course banquet. Especially when it's a Monday night and their favorite TV show is on in an hour.

Lengthy sex sessions It's not a myth that spiritual sex can go on for one or two hours. The reason isn't just sexual: it's to allow you to meditate as a couple with minimal movement to ensure an exchange of vital energies. In plain English, this still means he penetrates and you both stay locked together doing nothing much other than gazing into each other's eyes. Yes, it forces you to stay in the moment—but it doesn't guarantee you won't be bored silly.

Oral sex for her is ignored Despite emphasizing again and again how important it is for the woman to be fully aroused before penetration, there's scant reference to the technique which gives most women their orgasms. Surely a sin punishable by death?

high-energy swing

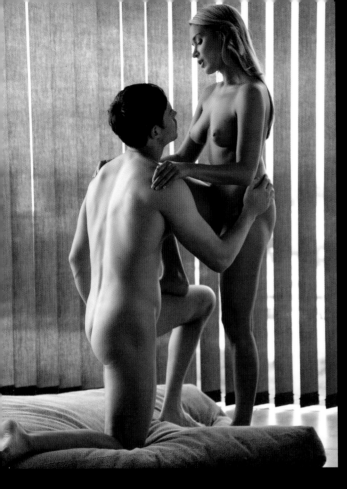

<< STEP ONE

Stand facing each other. He then drops to one knee, as though he's about to propose. She lifts the same side leg as his high knee and places her foot, gently, on the top of his thigh, nestling into his hip bone. Her toes point out with her heel facing inward. This is the moment when you gaze intently into each other's eyes, connecting emotionally before you move on to more physical stuff.

STEP TWO

Enough gazing, you're now ready for some saucy stuff. She lowers herself onto his thigh, putting her arms around his neck for balance. He penetrates and you're both magically in position for a good, long erotic make out. If you're feeling more sinful than spiritual, throw in some breast fondling, too.

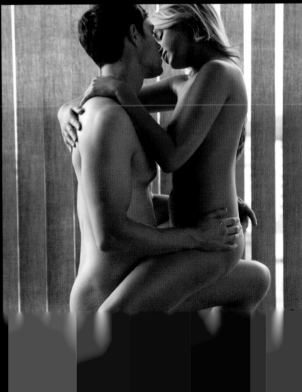

<< STEP THREE

Just when you were starting to relax, it all gets very high energy—well, for him anyway. She leans back, he grips her around the waist, pulling her pelvis close, while she holds onto his shoulders for support. He pulls her backward and forward in a small movement, but most of the work is done by her, as she internally squeezes and releases her vaginal muscles.

03

TOP POSITION

half-pressed

Elegant and balletic, this position looks splendidly choreographed but it is actually quite easy to do.

How to do it

She lies on her back and he kneels in front. Hanging onto his thighs for balance, she bends one knee, placing the sole of her foot on his chest, and stretches the other leg out as far as she can. He thrusts *carefully* (the angle is unusual, so experiment with shallow thrusting first).

Why you'd want to

It puts her clitoris in direct contact with his lower stomach. By rolling her pelvis, clitoral stimulation is pretty much guaranteed—and we all know clitoral orgasms are the easiest to come by (so to speak), so that's no small advantage!

Hot hint

If her leg starts to ache from being stretched out unsupported, think about how toned it'll look at the end of the session! Or you could position yourselves so she can put it against a wall and take a (well-deserved) rest.

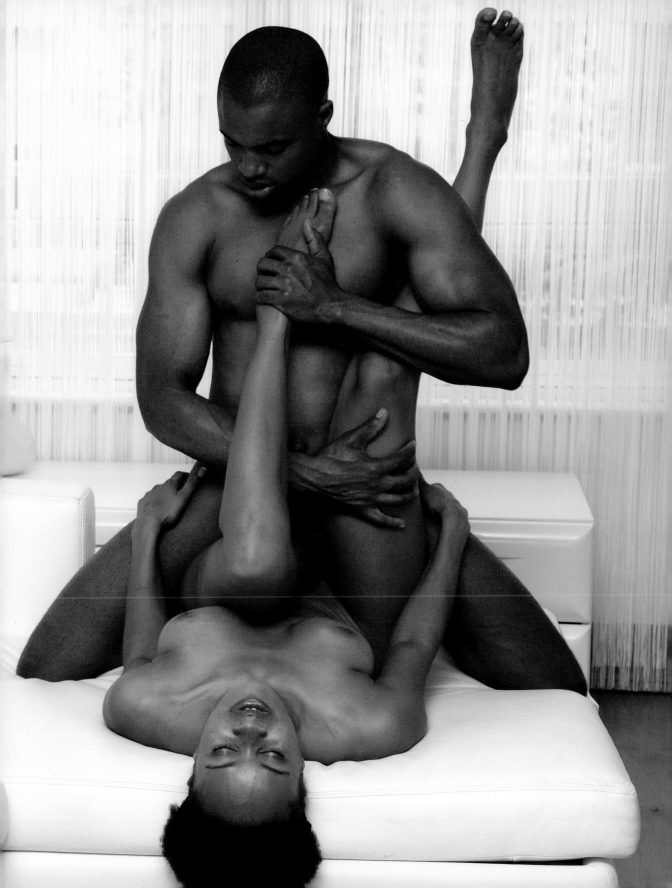

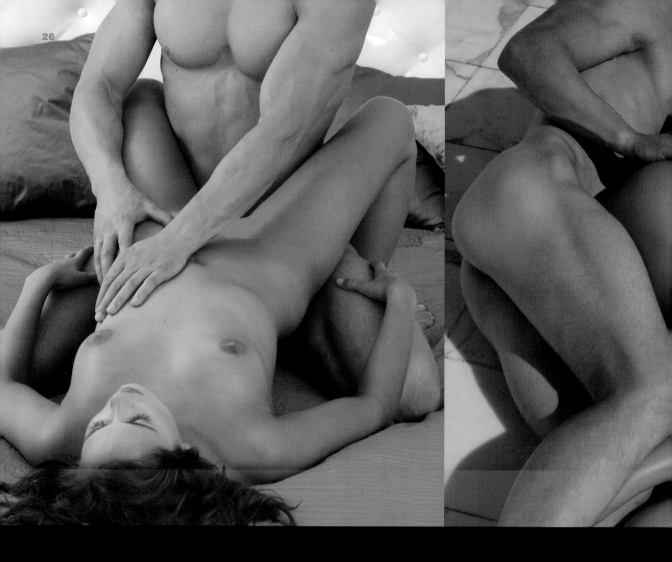

Sex for a snuggly, cuddly Sunday

START WITH THE LAZY BONER THEN GIVE INTO SLEEPY SPOONS AFTER A LIQUID LUNCH. FEELING ENERGETIC AFTER A SNOOZE? HIPPY GIRL DOES THE TRICK!

LAZY BONER

This is a twist on the standard missionary position that makes it way more comfortable for him because he doesn't have to support his own weight on his elbows. Another bonus: he gets a fabulous view of her bod and complete control over his thrusting. She can vary the sensation on her end by opening her legs wide or wrapping them around his waist. For deep penetration, she can pull her knees up to her chin and put her feet on his shoulders.

SLEEPY SPOONS

Perfect for half-asleep-hungover Sunday morning sex, or post-boozy Sunday lunch sessions! This position is remarkably intimate, even though you're both facing in the same direction, because there's full body contact. He penetrates from behind, and she lifts her bottom and/or uses her hands to help him. He can kiss or bite her neck, easily reaching around to sneakily play with her breasts or clitoris. It's a great position, too, if she's pregnant!

HIPPY GIRL

She lies on her back and he kneels in front between her legs. She then lifts her bottom, allowing him to enter. He pulls her toward him, she reaches down to hold her ankles as he supports her by holding her hips. If she's flexible enough to take a firm hold, she can hold her legs open far wider. This is a good position if he has a big penis and she has a small vagina (don't worry, I won't tell if you won't). She's opened wide and by raising her hips, he's pushed deep inside.

rocking
horse

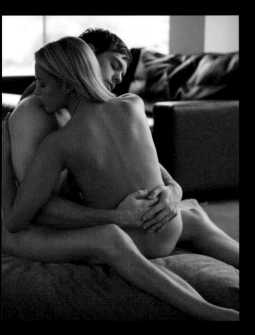

<< STEP ONE

He sits with legs stretched out, she sits sideways between his legs, with her legs over his thigh. Both hug and enjoy the flesh-to-flesh contact. There's no action yet but be patient: spiritual sex is as much about intimacy as it is passionate pounding!

STEP TWO

She provocatively places her ankle on his shoulder and holds her calf muscle. The point of this? Flexibility was seen as super-sexy! He's impressed by her sensual stretch *and* gets a view of her private parts, making
V him fully aroused.
V

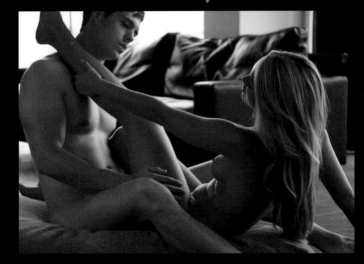

<< STEP FOUR

Clasp each other's wrists, then both lean backward, before moving into a rocking horse motion where one leans back as the other leans forward, pulling each other up with your arms. It's a sexual seesaw with the erotic focus on watching each other's faces as you experience pleasure.

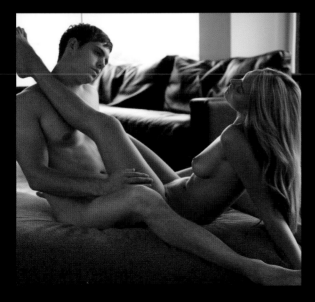

<< STEP THREE

He's—hurrah!—allowed to penetrate once she gives the secret signal and lets go of her leg. She leans back supporting her own weight, leaving one leg still on his shoulder and lifts her bottom to make it easier for him to enter. Don't attempt to thrust once you're in position, both simply enjoy the feel of his penis inside her vagina.

04

TOP POSITION

pressed

She lies back in a sexily submissive pose, giving him a fabulous bird's-eye view of the action.

How to do it
Moving on from the half-pressed position (see page 24), she now puts both feet against his chest, rather than just one, simultaneously hanging onto the top of his thighs to keep their groins pulled close. He holds onto her feet to hold her steady.

Why you'd want to
This position both shortens and tightens the vagina, making it a super-snug fit. It's also perfect for practicing any of the *Kama Sutra* or Tao thrusting techniques. Try the "sets of nine" (see page 153)—a mix of deep and shallow thrusts—for starters. An extra bonus: he has a prime view of his penis sliding in and out of her as he's performing.

Hot hint
This one's reasonably comfortable for both partners, though if she has extra long legs it might be a problem. (Nice one to have outside of bed though, so don't complain too vehemently!)

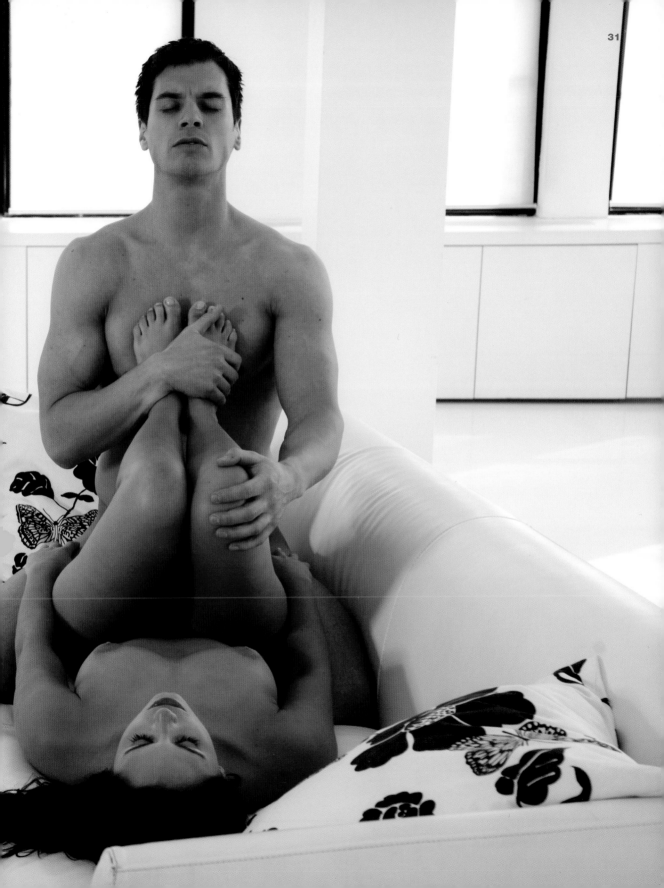

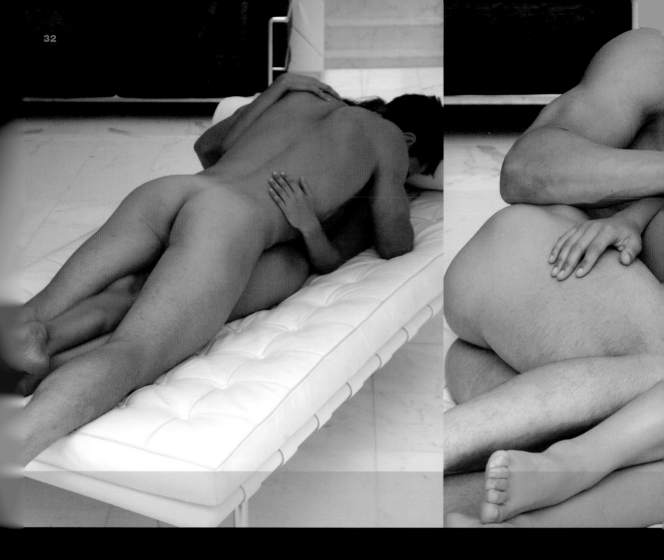

Three-way penetration plus

EACH OF THESE POSITIONS ALTERS THE ANGLE OF PENETRATION. EXPERIMENT IN ONE SINGLE, SUPERSEXY SESSION TO DISCOVER WHAT EXACTLY HITS THE SPOT.

THE ANKLE CROSS

This is a good one if his penis is on the small side: any position where she keeps her thighs pressed together rather than spread, keeps her tight and creates friction. Crossing her ankles keeps them in place during thrusting. Penetration is shallow—which has benefits for both of you. The first third of the vagina has the most nerve endings and it's the narrowest part of the canal, which guarantees him the tightest fit.

TIPSY SPOONS

It's a subtle variation on the sleepy spoons position and great for when you're both feeling slightly more awake. By her tipping on her side, turning her face and body to try to face him, the mood shifts from drowsy to raunchy. It's more involved, active love-making with both of you raised on your elbows rather than lying back. Add lots of rough kissing and neck biting and you've got a new favorite!

THE BENDOVER

It's an elegant version of rear entry which feels fabulous for both of you. He penetrates from behind, she leans forward, holding onto a piece of furniture for support. Crossing her ankles keeps things tantalizingly tight and by squeezing her vaginal and buttock muscles around his penis, she can up the sensation even further. It's versatile, too, since you don't really need props other than something for her to hold on to.

05

TOP POSITION

pressing

An easily achievable and intimate position which provides lovers with a sexy, skin-to-skin sensory treat

How to do it

You both start in the standard missionary position, she then bends her legs and presses her thighs around his body. This one's all about the action of gripping with the thighs—rather than just wrapping them around him— which has the effect of tightening both her vaginal and pelvic muscles. It's easily done by resting her calves on his lower back, ankles crossed, but it also works with her feet flat on the bed.

Why you'd want to

There's lots of lovely bodily contact for maximum skin stimulation and it's a twist on the old favorite: the missionary. Besides, sometimes it's nice for her that he's in a dominant position, completely pinning her down while she drapes herself around him.

Hot hint

If her thigh muscles tire, she can squeeze and release her pelvic floor muscles instead, "milking" his penis internally. It's a totally different sensation since his penis is being squeezed rather than "pulled" up and down.

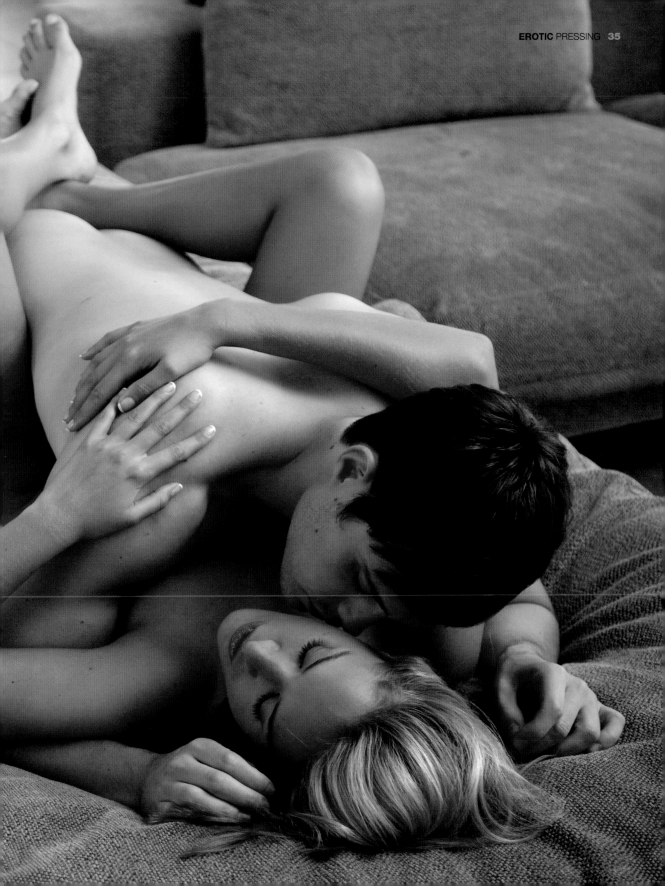

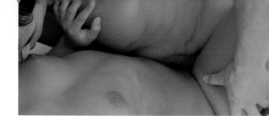

sex like it used to be

THE *KAMA SUTRA* SAYS FOREPLAY BEGINS WAY BEFORE THE FIRST TOUCH OR KISS. READ ON TO DISCOVER HOW TO FULLY PREPARE FOR SEX, THE IMPORTANCE OF LOOKING GOOD—AND A MASSAGE WITH MEANING.

The ancient Hindus were as body proud as they were hedonistic—Vatsyayana gives explicit and lengthy instructions on personal hygiene. A man should "bathe daily, anoint his body with oil every other day, apply a lathering substance to his body every three days, get his head shaved every four days, and the other parts of his body every five or ten days. All these things should be done without fail and the sweat of the armpits should also be removed." (Very good idea, that last suggestion.) On top of this, he should "put collyrium (an eye lotion) on his eyelids and below his eyes, color his lips with alacktaka (a dye), and look at himself in the glass." Yikes! Eye cream and lipstick—for boys! You can only guess at the lengthy beauty rituals women were in for!

Once both partners were suitably bathed and shaved, they would meet in the "pleasure room." This sumptuous sex pit was decorated with flowers, fragrant with perfume—and came with a fully stocked bar and hors d'oeuvres. Excellent! While eating and drinking "freely" (getting sloshed), the couple would carry on "amusing conversations" on various subjects (flirt) and might "also talk suggestively of things which would be considered as coarse" (talk dirty). When the lovers were "overcome with lust," the ever-present servants, who acted as waiters and waitresses, would discreetly disappear, and the couple would fall onto the bed.

If only sex was like that today. Well, apart from the servants waiting on you hand and foot, it can be! All Vatsyayana is describing is a sex session which has been planned, anticipated, and enjoyed. The sort of sex you had at the beginning of your relationship. Fact: people fall out of lust when sex is taken for granted. And they fall out of love if they're not having good, regular sex. If you want sex to be as good as it was at the start (and who doesn't?) give it and each other the same amount of attention you did then. It wasn't just hormones and the feel of fresh flesh, the sex was good because you gave it priority. Take a page out of the *Kama Sutra* and aim for at least one "special" sex session a month.

THINGS TO TRY

Make your bedroom sexy Keep it at the right temperature with low, flattering lighting (tea-light candles on plates on the floor work well). Burn oils or scented candles, put some music on. The *Kama Sutra* encourages you to involve all five senses in sex—not just touch and sight.

Make yourselves sexy Vatsyayana recognized the importance of looking good for your partner, so get yourselves out of those sweatpants and slide into something less comfortable—and sexier!

Have some "treat" nibbles in bed Eat these and have a glass of bubbly either before or after sex.

Have a bath together Soap each other's bodies and dry each other off afterward.

Wash each other's hair Lots of people find this sexy, particularly if it involves a nice head massage. Others find shampoo in their eyes and running eye makeup from water all over their face, not so hot.

Give each other a massage Yes, yes you've heard this a billion times before… so why don't you do it! Massages, like kissing, tend to happen at the start, then peter out rapidly. Resurrect them (see right).

Play beauty therapist Face massages are just as relaxing as body massages, albeit a little less sexy. Make sure their skin is nice and clean (use cleanser and damp cotton balls first), then, using almond oil, put their head in your lap and make slow, relaxing circles on their face, using both hands. Slide your hands under their neck, massaging the top of their shoulders by making fists with your hands.

Brush or play with each other's hair Rather handily, you can do this one while watching TV.

Give each other a foot massage—then do naughty things with your toes. Explicit illustrations of *Kama Sutra* positions often showed men using their big toe on the clitoris to satisfy more than one woman simultaneously. Do it under the tablecloth next time you're at a fancy restaurant (though it's probably best to stick with just your partner rather than include the woman at the next table).

MASSAGE WITH A MESSAGE

Turn a standard body massage into a meaningful one by focusing on the seven energy centers in your partner's body. Tantrics call these "chakras"—little power generators which sit in different parts of your body, creating and storing energy for you. The idea behind all that breathing, pelvic bouncing, and fire breathing (just a few of the fun things Tantrics get up to) is to open up these energy centers so the *kundalini* (energy) can move freely throughout your body. Sexual energy is particularly potent which is why Tantrics are so sex crazy. Today we're taught to focus our energy and attention on the genitals during orgasm, Tantra teaches you to do the opposite and move it away to the rest of your body. Tantrics mentally focus on each chakra but stroking and/or massaging the area feels great, too. I know, I know, normally I go *blah!* at the soppy stuff but explaining what each chakra is responsible for during a massage can be quite a bonding experience.

The base/root chakra is at the base of the spine, just above the perineum (between the genitals and anus). This one governs our instincts and genetic coding.

The pelvic/sacral chakra is at the genitals. This governs our sexual life.

The naval/solar plexus chakra is at the navel. It governs our personal power.

The heart chakra is at the heart and, predictably, governs our love.

The throat chakra governs communication.

The brow/forehead chakra is between the brows. It governs our intellect and thought processes.

The crown chakra is at the crown of the head and the home of the goddess Shakti (and you thought the voices in your head meant you were crazy!) The god Shiva lives in the brow chakra. People try to move their energy from the base chakra to the brow and then to the crown to free Shiva and reunite him with Shakti. Known as "enlightenment," we call it "The Mother of all Orgasms" since that's what it's supposed to produce.

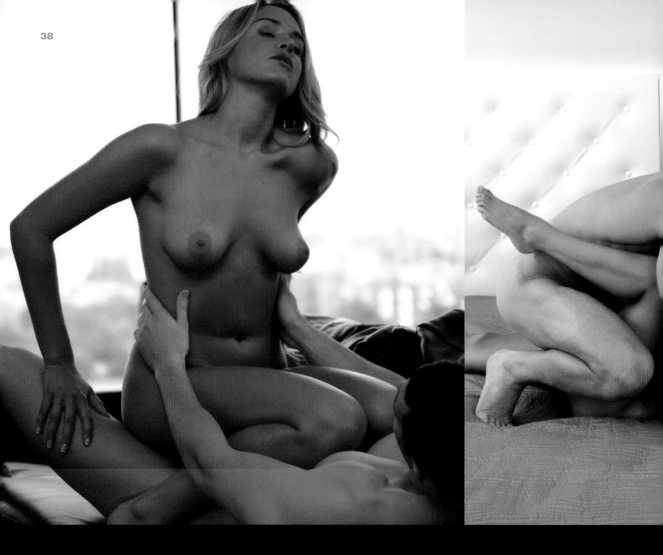

Tackle some take-turns sex

THIS THREE-WAY SEQUENCE ALTERS THE MOOD ALONG WITH THE POSITION, MIXING THINGS UP NICELY FOR A SESSION TO REMEMBER.

THE BEE

Feeling particularly strong? Try the bee. It looks deceptively easy, but you need both strength and practice to master it. He lies on his back and she jumps on top, feet flat on the bed beside his hips then, holding his knees for support and leverage, swings her hips both left and right over his penis, hovering in sensual circles, just as a bee floats above a flower. It's all about varying her hip movements to produce exquisite sensations for both of you.

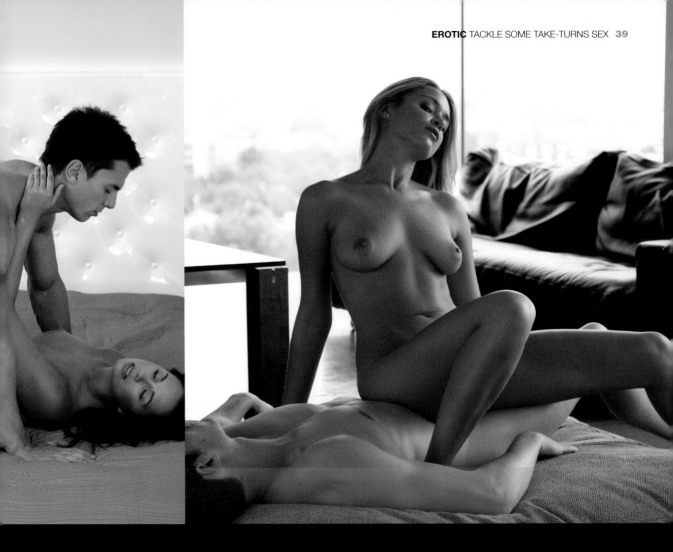

SEXUAL EQUALITY

He flips her over onto her back and takes control. He needs good balance and you both need a relatively coordinated rhythm for this position, but it's worth making the effort because it puts both the penis and vagina in alignment. He usually enters with a downward thrust, so this is a deliciously different spin on penetration. Simple changes—like him squatting instead of lying with legs outstretched—dramatically affect

SENSUAL SWAN

She's still on top but sitting side-saddle, which alters the angle of the vagina, providing a fresh, new feeling for both of you. Granted it's hard for her to move but *he* can, by pushing up his hips. Instead, she sits back and looks beautiful in this body-flattering pose. It's called "the swan" because this position is graceful and reminiscent of a swan gliding elegantly

elephant

Animalistic, primitive, and positioned to hit super-sensitive spots, this one puts him in charge of her pleasure.

How to do it

If you're looking for new, exciting ways to make love, look no further than the animal kingdom, says Vatsyayana perceptively. This position is inspired by the mating of elephants (except you won't have to laboriously mount with a penis that literally weighs a ton!) She lies on her front on the bed, pressing her thighs together, rather than apart. She can lift her upper torso off the bed to get closer to him or lie flat. He penetrates from behind, supporting his weight on his arms, straddling the outside of her thighs.

Why you'd want to

Rear-entry positions are fantastic for fantasizing because you can pretend your partner is whoever you want him or her to be! There's no clitoral stimulation for her, but he'll hit the sensitive front vaginal wall so there's more chance of a vaginal/G-spot orgasm.

Hot hint

The higher she tilts her bottom, the more directly he'll hit the front vaginal wall.

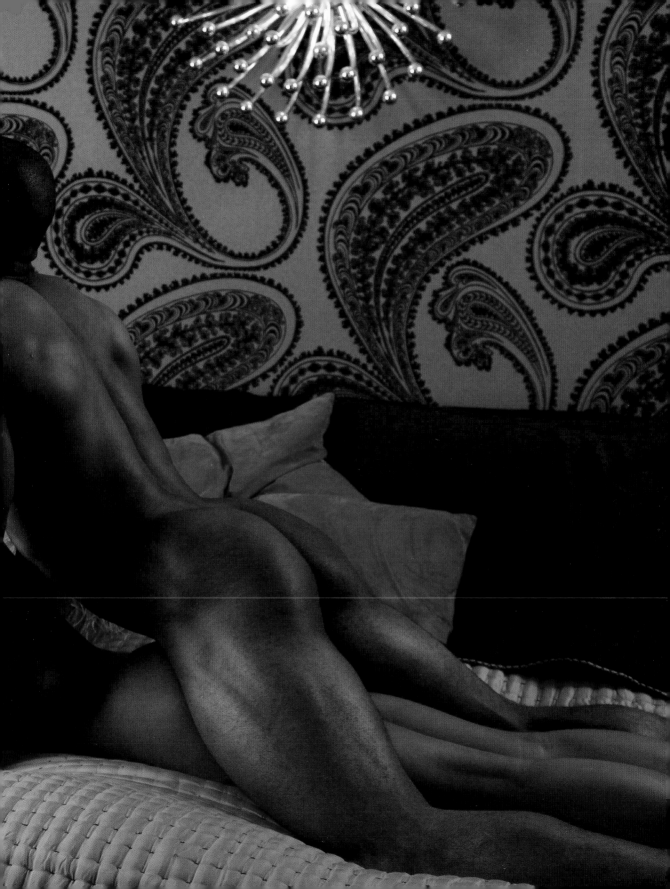

rear view

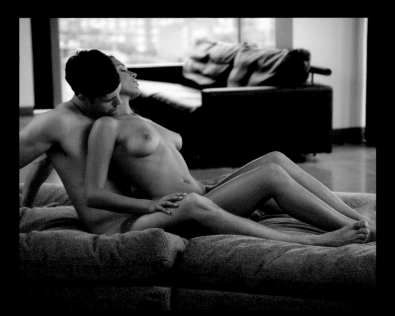

<< STEP ONE

He lies back on the bed, legs stretched out and apart, and supports his weight on his outstretched arms. She lies back against his chest and pushing back against him for leverage, lifts her bottom and uses her hands to help him penetrate before settling into his lap and relaxing against him.

>> STEP TWO

By alternately arching her back, then relaxing back against him, she creates enough friction to stimulate both of them. He's in a prime position to nibble her neck and whisper horribly filthy things into her ear—or sweet soulful somethings, which is probably more what Vatsyayana intended!

<< STEP THREE

Squeezing her legs together, she leans forward and puts her hands on her ankles to hold herself there. (The truly flexible will put palms flat on the floor.) This squeezes his penis. He, meanwhile, clenches his thighs around her buttock cheeks as both rock to and fro. For men who sometimes (OK, often) enjoy watching her bottom rather than her face, this could become a sexy staple!

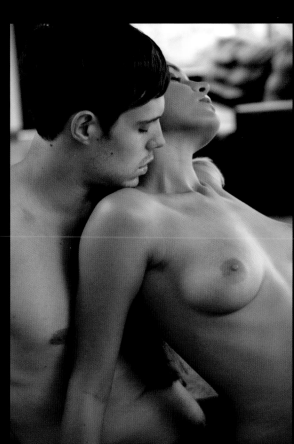

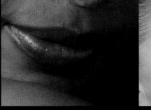
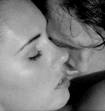

kiss-ass kissing

IT'S NOT JUST A CASE OF LOCKING LIPS: TRY THE THROBBING KISS, THE BENT KISS, INDULGE IN A BIT OF TONGUE FIGHTING—AND TRY OUT THE TECHNIQUE RUMORED TO MAKE A WOMAN CLIMAX PURELY BY KISSING.

The *Kama Sutra* turns kissing into an art form. It doesn't just tell you how to kiss (in painstaking detail), it tells you where, when, and what type of kiss to use if you want to do everything from wake your partner for morning sex. "The kiss that kindles love" involves planting one on them while they're sleeping to show you're in the mood for sex) to how to annoy the hell out of them ("the kiss that turns away" is what you do when you're feeling needy and they're not paying enough attention to you). Kissing is seen as a powerful tool to manipulate your lover and get your needs met. Want a bit? A woman who places her head on a man's thigh while bathing him, then gives a little kiss on the thigh, has landed "a demonstrative kiss" designed to "inflame" him. There are lots of fancy names for standard smackers as well. All of which sound extremely exotic—but most actually aren't! The "throbbing" kiss, for instance, is simply a kiss where you move the lower lip but not the top one. The "bent" kiss sounds magnificently kinky, but in fact means your faces are at an angle to each other. "Tongue fighting" is simply our version of French kissing.

But it's the kissing games which are the most amusing. One involves her waiting until her lover's asleep, then grabbing hold of his lower lip in her teeth. Which sounds quite sexy—until you read the next part: she's then supposed to be "laughing and making a loud noise, deriding him, and dancing around, saying whatever she likes in a joking way, while moving her eyebrows and rolling her eyes." Clearly what got the ancient Indians going years ago wouldn't quite cut it today.

In Hindu and Tantric texts, the kiss is also considered a big deal because they believe mingling saliva harmonizes the opposite energies of men and women. It's so sacred and intimate in India, until recently, kissing wasn't even shown in films and husband and wife would never pucker up publicly. Even today, we can't hide how up-close and personal kissing is. Sex workers often refuse to do it and it's still one of the most intimate ways lovers communicate with each other. Here's what the mystical masters have to say about making mouth music.

CLEVER KISSING TECHNIQUES WORTH TAKING

Considering the tongue contains more nerves and muscles than almost any other part of the body, it's not hard to figure out why tongue-tussling features strongly in our sexuality today. Happily, it plays a key role in spiritual sex as well. Combine lots of tongue action with some rather creative sucking techniques and bucket loads of intense gazing and you're on the way to Tantric kiss bliss!

The *uttarachumbita* Weird name—weird concept. But massively appealing! Tantrics believe there's a direct link between the clitoris and a woman's upper lip—to the point where he can actually give her an orgasm without ever removing her panties! See if it works for you two. First, get her to lift her top lip, look above her two front teeth and find the small piece of connective tissue between her upper lip and her gum. That's the frenulum—the bit you needs to focus on. Start kissing with you sucking her top lip, while she sucks on your bottom one. Using your tongue, find her frenulum and suck and draw on it using your tongue and lips. She didn't feel any tingling down below? Never mind—it still feels pretty damn sexy!

The eye lock Make loads of eye contact during kissing and you add both intimacy and eroticism.

The yucky breathe-in-each-other's-breath one Yes, I have previously dismissed this as stomach turning gross but... if you can get past the thought of it (and happen to be involved with someone with fresh breath), it actually does make you feel much closer. Press your foreheads together for a minute or more, then have a conventional kiss, except inhale while they're exhaling and vice versa. As they breathe out, you're breathing in. As you do it, imagine you're giving yourself to each other through your breath. I know, it still sounds silly, but just try it once.

Soul kissing This is an incredibly intimate and bonding exercise so best save it for a long-term lover rather than a bit on the side. Get your partner to masturbate to orgasm while you kiss them intensely and erotically. Then, as you feel them about to climax, pull back, get them to open their eyes and hold their face in your hands looking deep into their eyes.

AND THERE'S MORE...

Suck their tongue, lick the inside of their lips, nip their lips with your teeth.

Use your tongue to explore their whole face—lick their eyelids, ears, and underside of the chin. Sounds yucky? Think about the other parts of them you happily lick!

Suck each other's tongues simultaneously—hard—when you're both on the verge of orgasm.

Insert your fingers as you lick and suck on their mouth, and let them suck on them as well.

Use your tongue to explore their hands—the skin between the fingers is particularly sensitive. Pushing your tongue in between them has connotations of cunnilingus; sucking his thumb conjures up delicious thoughts of what you might move on to do to his penis…

Keep kissing erotically after either of you orgasm and you're much more likely to keep going and enjoy seconds.

Flick your tongue up underneath their top lip, tug on their bottom lip with your teeth.

Lick the roof of their mouth—some people love this, others—like me—find that it just tickles and feels really weird!

Thrust with your tongue, imitating intercourse, while you're having it.

Pull back between kisses to read their expression and make eye contact. When they impatiently lunge back in, hold back for a few seconds to tease.

To make a kiss soulful, cradle their face in your hands, to make it passionate hold their arms above their hand with one hand, and explore their body with your other while you kiss.

carnal
cuddle

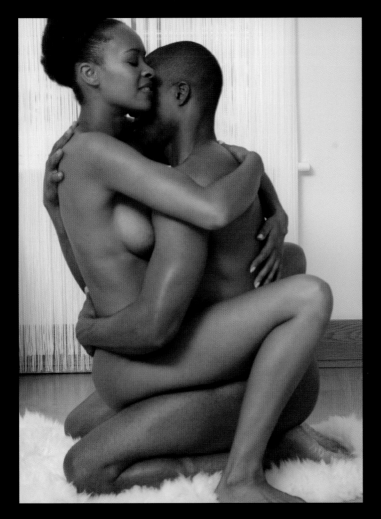

<< STEP ONE

He kneels on a hard surface, legs tucked beneath him. She climbs on top, positioning herself high on his thighs so she's riding him. Both hug closely for balance and to keep him penetrated. She can experiment by moving higher or lower on his thighs to hit the most sensitive spot on her vaginal wall. She's got several? Well who's a lucky girl?

<< STEP TWO

Move into a rocking motion and you set off a subtle but exquisitely effective thrusting sensation. Her feet are flat on the floor giving her something to push against. He lifts up on his thighs. It's way easier if he keeps his back erect and his stomach muscles turned on. (Yes, you can skip the gym tomorrow.) It's easy to do— and easy for her to keep him hard by squeezing her pelvic floor muscles.

erotic

exotic

exhilarating

exhibitionist

expert

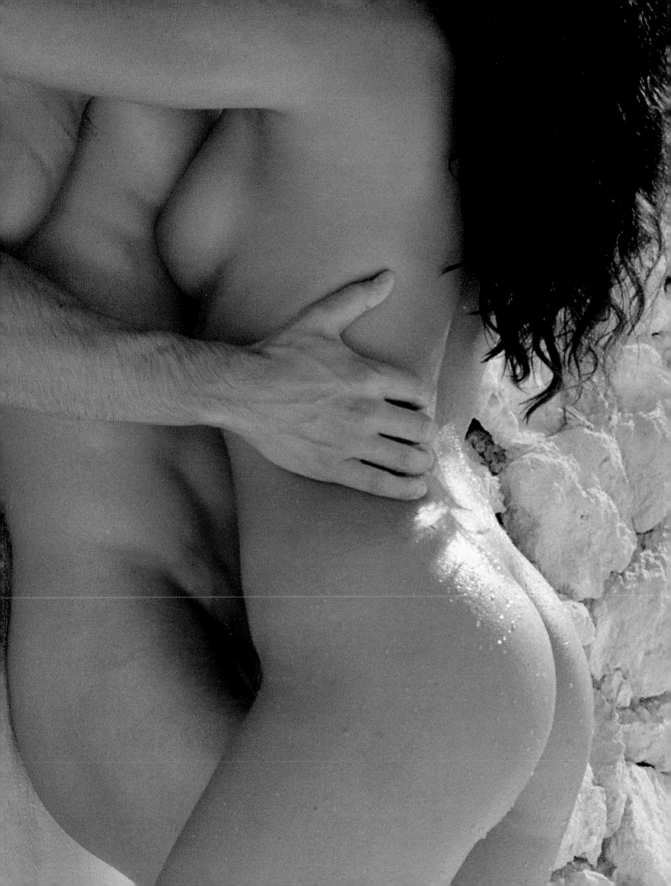

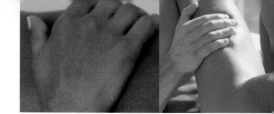

exotic, erotic embraces and quirky ways to court

EMBRACES LOOM LARGE IN SPIRITUAL SEX, RANGING FROM THE TENDER "TOUCHING" TO MORE ARDENT VARIETIES LIKE THE "PRESSING" EMBRACE (SIMPLY SLAM THEM AGAINST A WALL!). THE QUESTION IS: WILL TWINING LIKE A CREEPER AND CLIMBING TREES GET YOU ANYWHERE TODAY?

Thoroughness and formalized rituals: it's the very core of the *Kama Sutra* that most modern people grapple with. Why such relentless detail for such simple things—like an embrace? Well, Vatsyayana saw life as something to be understood and mastered, which ultimately meant taking everything apart and examining all the elements to figure out how it all worked. To him, a hug isn't just a hug, it sends a myriad of signals to both participants. After analyzing celebrity couple's body language for years—based heavily on hugs (or the lack of them)—I have to say, I heartily agree. An embrace is never just an embrace—there is a message in each and every one of them. Tentative and charged: By God I desire you. Warm and close: I love you. Stiff and distant: I'm angry with you. Has our snuggling and cuddling style changed over the past, ohh 2,000 years? Surprisingly, less than you think: there *are* lessons to be learned. I've put eight embraces to the test on the opposite page.

WOULD IT WORK TODAY?

Just how many of the other ancient courtship rituals would work in today's world? More than you'd expect! (These were all originally intended for him to use on her, by the way, but these days advances are made by both sexes, so I've made them unisex.)

✔ *Describe to them the pangs you suffer on their account.* Just don't get too soppy too soon.

✔ *At parties, sit near them, place your foot on theirs and slowly touch each of their toes.* An oldie but a goodie—playing footsie can be incredibly sexy.

✔ *Whenever you give anything to them or take anything from them, show by your manner and look how much you love them.* Intense face gazing and eye contact still works great today.

✗ *Tell them about a beautiful dream you've had about someone else attractive.* Guaranteed to backfire—big time!

✗ *Vatsyayana says it's just "talk" that women grow "less timid than usual during the evening and in darkness and are more desirous of sex at those times."* He clearly wasn't a drinker. Everyone knows females are much more likely to have a wine (or two or six) after 6 pm and that inhibitions lower, along with the buttons on her top…

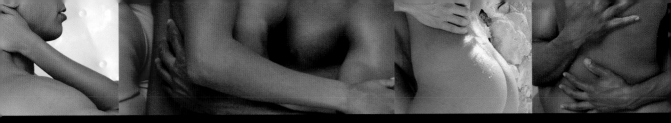

THE EIGHT EMBRACES

I'm crazy about you, but haven't worked up the courage to tell you...

The touching embrace He "accidentally" brushes up against her and touches her on the front or the side.
Today: Lust-struck lovers often deliberately put their hands, thighs, or feet close to a longed-for person and pretend a touch was accidental. You can definitely try this one at home.

The piercing embrace She bends over, as if to pick something up from the ground, her breasts touch him, and he fondles them.
Today: Better tone this one down a tad. Fondling breasts before actually asking someone out isn't done (except in a fantasy). Caress with eyes only.

You're officially dating, but haven't done the deed yet...

The rubbing embrace You're out strolling in public and your bodies rub up against each other.
Today: Nothing new there then.

The pressing embrace Overcome by lust, one of you pushes the other up against a wall or pillar.
Today: Pillars might be short in supply, but fridges work just as well.

You're just about to do it...

Twining like a creeper Standing, she clings closely, like a vine to a tree, pulls his face down to hers, and looks lovingly at him, desperate to be kissed.

Today: Do this and he'll be kissing your face off in a matter of seconds.

Like climbing a tree Standing, she places one foot on the man's foot and the other foot on his thigh, one arm around his back and the other around his neck, sighing and cooing.
Today: Definitely not to be done in public or if you've already got a bit of reputation as a slight nut case. This could confirm it. Instead, lift one leg and wrap it around his thigh while doing the arm stuff. Sighing and cooing is optional.

You're doing it...

Mixing sesame seeds with rice Lying down hugging closely in a tangle or arms and legs, rubbing thighs together.
Today: Standard feverish behavior—though we call it by a less romantic name (humping).

Like water in milk: You're both so in love, there's no such thing as pain or discomfort as your bodies squeeze so close together, you could be melting into each other. Can be done lying or with her sitting in his lap.
Today: *Awwwww* or vomit, depending on whether you're the romantic type.

And if you get bored with those...

Embrace just a part of each other's body by simply pressing or gently touching your body part to theirs... try your thighs, breasts, and forehead.

An embrace is never just an embrace—there is a message in each and every one of them! Tentative and charged: by God I desire you. Warm and close: I love you.

07

TOP POSITION

side-by-side

Face-to-face, intense eye contact, snuggled in each other's arms… this is more like an erotic cuddle than full-blown sex.

How to do it

A fantastic position to introduce a reluctant lover to spiritual sex, this one is dead easy to master. Start in the good old missionary position—him on top—then once he's penetrated, roll onto your sides, wrapping your arms around each other for support, his thigh straddling her hip. Don't attempt conventional thrusting here, instead squeeze those pelvic floor muscles and enjoy more subtle thrusting movements.

Why you'd want to

Her thighs are together, which makes her feel tantalizingly tight. And when you're done with the soulful stuff, it's perfect for talking dirty face-to-face. Had a rough day at the office? Side-by-side is perfect for moments when you feel more languid than lusty.

Hot hint

This one's so ridiculously easy and armchair comfy, you don't need any hints to get it right! Enjoy the comfort while it lasts (you wait until you get to chapter five!)

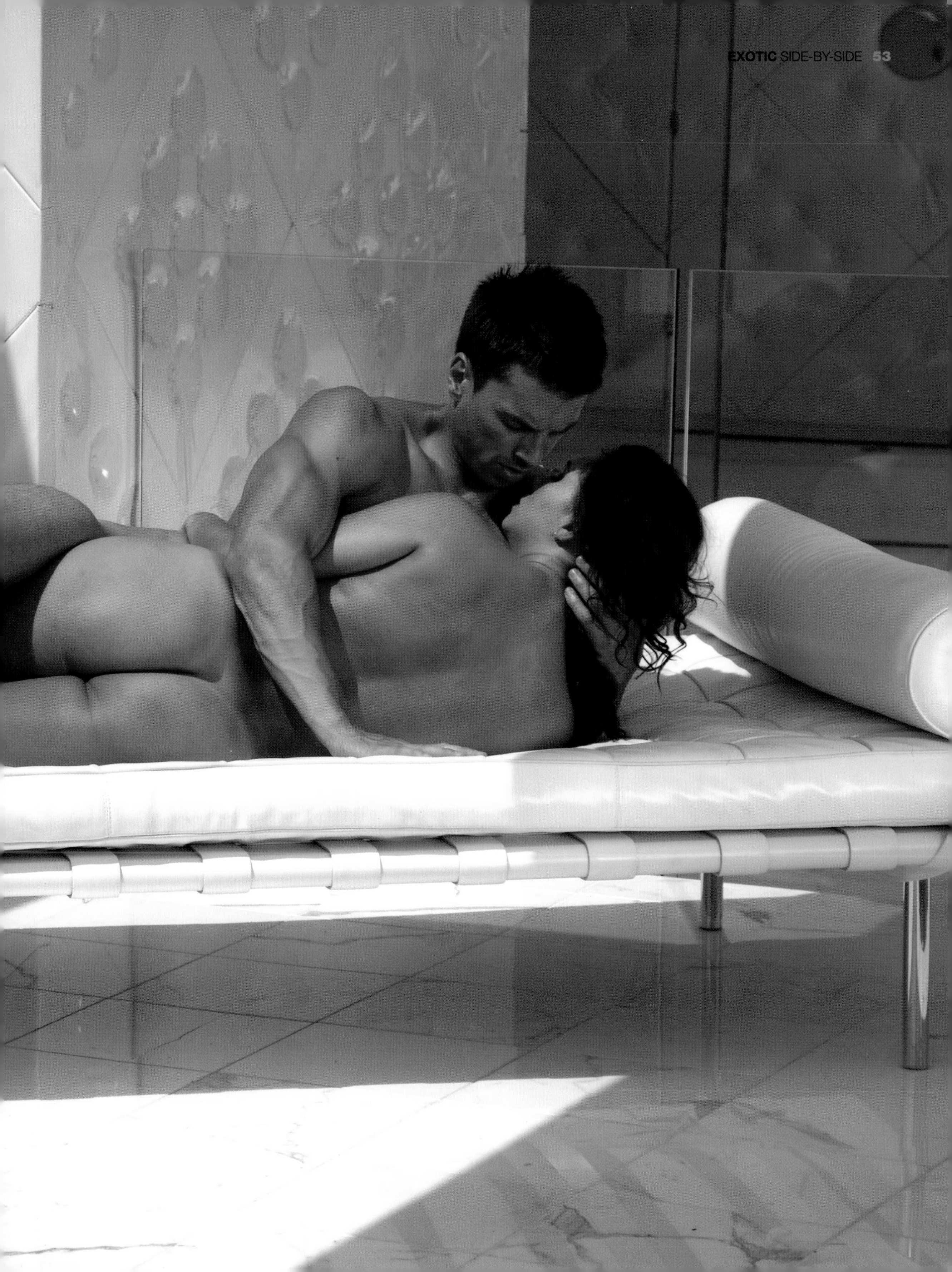

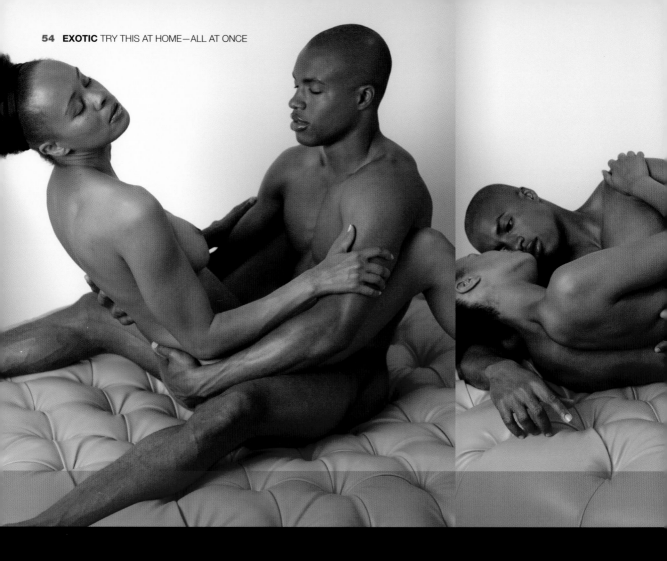

Try this at home—all at once

THIS IS A FABULOUS SEQUENCE IF YOU WANT TO MOVE SEAMLESSLY FROM WOMAN ASTRIDE TO A SIDEWAYS POSITION, AND THEN BACK AGAIN.

LOVERS' LINK

He sits with legs extended and apart. She lowers herself on top, allowing him to penetrate, before sitting on his lap. She clasps his upper arms, he supports her back. This pose isn't actually intended to provide an orgasm for each of you, rather a relaxing way to simply enjoy being sexually linked. Again, it's all about appreciating each sexual feeling for its own worth rather than thinking all roads lead to intercourse. (Bet you can't do it without wiggling!)

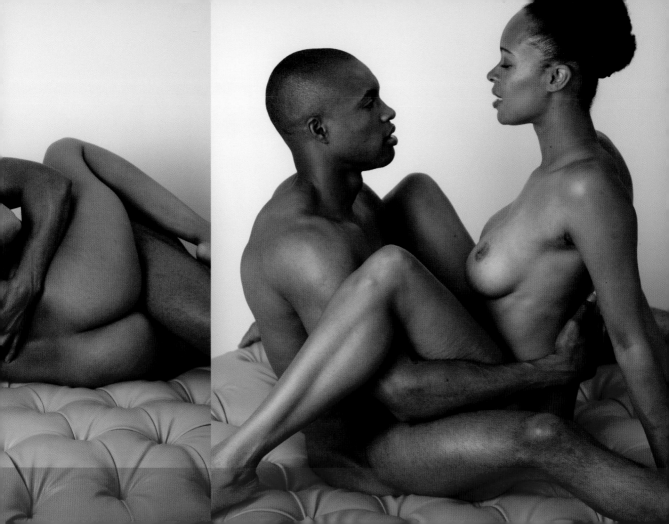

08

TOP POSITION

clasping

If this looks familiar, that's because it is! It's another name for the old faithful, the missionary position.

How to do it

When you like getting up close and personal, you can't beat just climbing on top! Which is basically what's happening here: she lies flat on her back with legs apart, he jumps on top and enters and—*voila!*—you've just

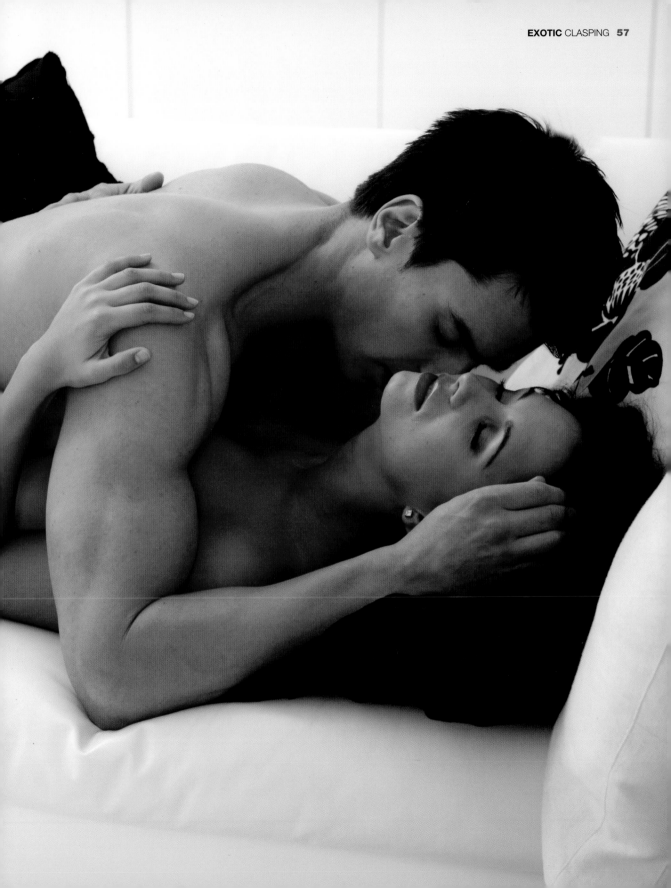

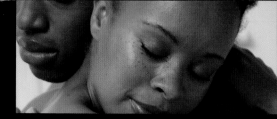

sex with soul

MODERN SOCIETY TENDS TO SEPARATE SEX AND LOVE—SPIRITUAL SEX WORKS ON REUNITING THE TWO. IF YOU'D LIKE SEX WHICH MERGES RAUNCH AND ROMANCE, YOU'VE COME TO THE RIGHT PLACE!

There's a moment during orgasm when the rest of the world around you ceases to exist. For those precious few seconds, you are 100 percent truly, utterly, and exclusively concentrated on what you are experiencing. Simultaneously immersed, drowning, floating in pleasure. Now just imagine if you could make that feeling last almost the *entire* time you are having sex—and your partner is in that bubble with you.

That's soul sex.

Want some? Thought you might. Thing is, while we like to pretend we're fascinated purely by the exotic positions in the *Kama Sutra*, it's also because it hints at a different type of sex—sex which is a hell of a lot better than what we're currently having. Plenty of people feel disappointed by their sex lives. Sex and spirituality are poles apart today. We pride ourselves on being realists and are encouraged to think about things we can prove and touch, rather than intangibles. We wouldn't want to be seen as fanciful now, would we? A dreamer. Have our head in the clouds. Spiritual sex requires a completely different type of thinking than we're used to… but still, it remains sort of tempting. As Deepak Chopra, undisputed king of mind-body medicine, says, "Even those who hunger for pleasures of the flesh are actually seeking the soul in disguise." Just as falling in love lifts us above the mundanity of real life, sending us on a vacation in enjoyable madness, the thought that sex could do the same—and not just in the beginning but for a lifetime—is damn appealing.

Changing your attitude to achieve this takes time, but the key elements to doing it are easy to grasp: reacquaint those old friends love and sex and give your love life the most precious gift we have in today's modern world: time.

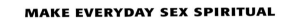

MAKE EVERYDAY SEX SPIRITUAL

These are small but significant ways you can turn wham-bam-thank-you-maam sex into something with a little more depth and feeling.

Stop thinking of sex as a physical activity

Instead think of it as a way of connecting your minds and souls as well as your bodies.

Imagine you're exchanging energy Even if you honestly don't believe you can move sexual energy around your body at will (see page 13), you can't argue with the concept of it. It's really just another term to describe arousal and feeling turned on.

Maintain eye contact during sex Most of us close our eyes during sex to concentrate on the sensations of what's happening to our body. Others do it because they feel faintly embarrassed looking at each other, convinced a fit of the giggles is a heartbeat away. It *does* feel a bit weird and overly intimate at the start, but once you get past the initial discomfort it's deeply sexy and you *do* feel a lot more connected. If you can't maintain contact the whole way through, take baby steps and try it for short bursts of time. (You're supposed to continue the "eye lock" during kissing. But if you're like me, seeing two eyes weirdly morph into one is likely to spark musings of alien invasions rather than tender thoughts!).

Match your breathing While exchanging breaths—you inhale what they're exhaling and vice versa – doesn't appeal to the squeamish (or sensible, if it's the morning after the night before and he's had garlic bread and beer), breathing in time is simple and effective. It's calming, slows you down, and does make you feel more "as one."

Have sex without a goal Stop judging the success of your sessions by how many or how intense your orgasms were or how many positions you tried. Stop thinking of sex as having a beginning (foreplay), a middle (intercourse), and an end (orgasm). Instead, think of it as a time when you're going to pleasure each other and be connected.

Be present in the moment This isn't just a spiritual sex rule—it's something almost all therapists get couples to work on. It's way, way too easy during sex to let the voices in your head hijack you: "Yuk, look at the dimpling on my thigh!/Is she enjoying this? Bet her ex was better at it/Jesus Christ, is that the time? The kids are going to be home any minute. And what the hell will I give them for dinner? Maybe I should defrost something from the freezer..." While you're mentally reaching for the fish fingers, your poor partner's killing themselves, trying to come up with the carnal equivalent of Beethoven's Fifth with whatever part they've got their hands, tongue, bits attached to. During sex, try to stop thinking and start feeling. Be in the room, in the now. Do this by keeping your eyes open and focused on what's happening. Concentrate on all your senses: what you are smelling, feeling, seeing, hearing. If you feel your thoughts pulling you away, drag yourself back.

Don't equate speed with passion At times you'll want to dispense with the niceties, rip each other's clothes off, and have furious, frenzied, lusty sex. I'm not suggesting for a moment that you don't (God forbid!), just that you stop thinking of those sessions as the "hot" ones and slower, more soulful sex as the "romantic" version. Sex slowed up can be unbearably, tortuously erotic. It just means paying attention to more subtle sensations. Looking in, a couple doing Kabazzah, a Tantric technique, won't appear to be having much fun. He's inside her, but they're completely still with no movement from the waist down. What you can't see is her "milking" him—squeezing her pelvic floor muscles to massage his penis. While I'm a huge fan of quick sex, there's a biological reason to slow sex down. Touch and arousal sets off the secretion of natural hormones. Some sexologists believe quick sex isn't emotionally satisfying because there's not enough time for these to be released into the bloodstream. The postcoital "feel-good" factor is short-circuited.

cocoon

<< STEP ONE

Simply hug, breathing in unison and appreciating each other. It's supposed to be a gentle "let's connect on a spiritual level" one, but you can heat things up by kissing (see page 45). Stay in the moment, at least for a few minutes, before moving on to step two.

STEP TWO

He kneels, she climbs on top, continuing to cuddle. He's now inside her, but no thrusting just yet! This is all about merging as one, so you both feel "cocooned" in your love for each other. Soppy, yes, but come on— there's penetration so it's not in that "We have to talk" category. Just stay still and be patient!

<< STEP THREE

Now you can move on to some real action…She leans back and he lifts her high off the bed and onto his thighs. She hangs onto his neck for support as he begins moving her back and forth to create some much-longed for friction. Move in close again if you like continuing the kissing (and who doesn't).

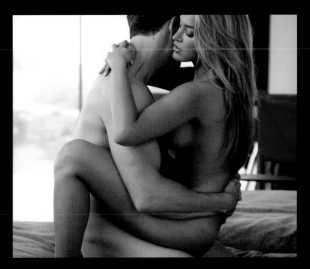

09

TOP POSITION

highest yawning

The unusual entry angle of this position provides a feisty, fresh start for a sensational session in the sack.

How to do it

She lies on her back and lifts her legs up and back toward her head. He kneels in front and penetrates, leaning his hips against her bottom cheeks for support, while she rests her calves on his shoulders and hangs onto his bottom cheeks.

Why you'd want to

Lifting her legs so high, simultaneously narrows her vagina and allows him to plunge incredibly deep. Vary the pace and intensity by switching between fast and shallow strokes and deep, slow ones.

Hot hint

Not a great choice if you've just had a romantic but rich three-course dinner! Her legs pressing against a full stomach can have the unfortunate reaction of producing, well, gas. If you feel rumblings in the wrong places, delicately put one leg down on the bed, then follow with the other. Better still switch to a far safer side-by-side position and save this for an empty stomach time!

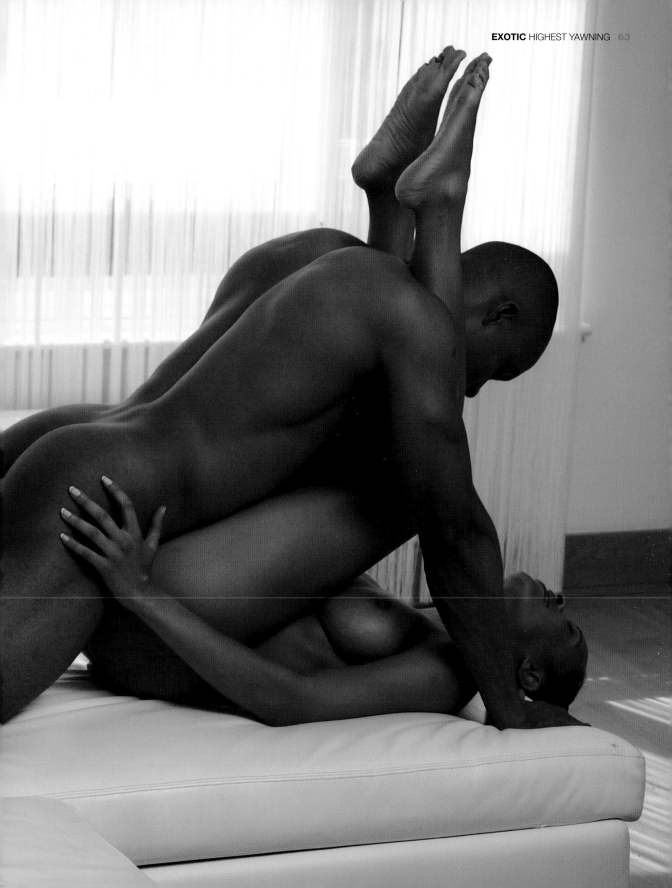

Laid-back poses for lazy lovers

WANT A LITTLE, BUT AREN'T QUITE UP TO ENERGETIC SEXUAL ACROBATICS? THESE THREE POSITIONS OFFER LOW-EFFORT, HIGH-STIMULATION SOLUTIONS.

RANDY ROBOT

This looks odd for several reasons. First, it's unusual for her to lie flat on top of him—she would normally sit up. But that's not nearly as odd as her holding her arms by her sides in such a robotic fashion. (Like, if you don't feel like it, just say so!). The *Kama Sutra* suggests she lies in this way because it puts her in the steering position. I have to be honest, this isn't exactly a runaway favorite because it can feel dispassionate. Others get off on that very fact: forbidding each other to get turned on can have the opposite effect!

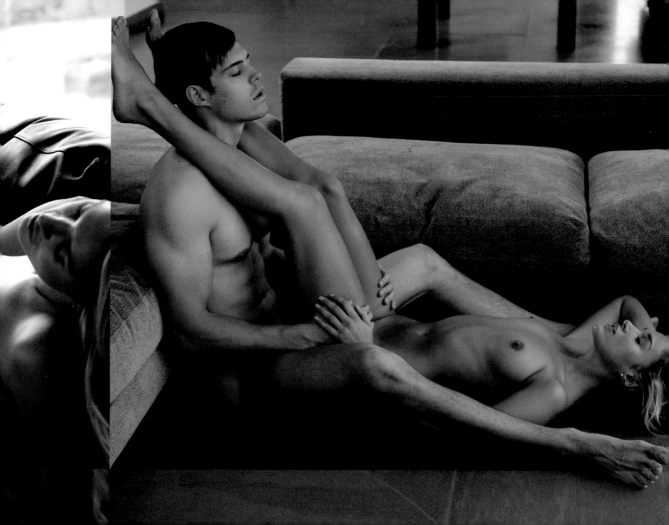

butterfly

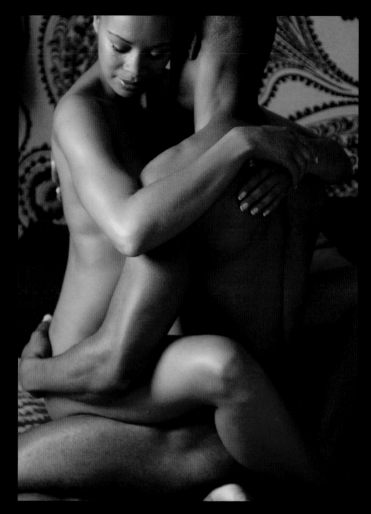

<< STEP ONE

He kneels with legs bent underneath him, she climbs onto his lap and the two of you embrace. He penetrates right from the start, but no naughty thrusting just yet! Yes, you're sensing a theme here—the idea is to draw things out rather than rush straight into it. Savor the moment.

STEP TWO

She starts to gently move up and down on his penis, but it's her pelvic floor muscles that are doing the main work, rather than her thighs. By quickly and repetitively squeezing and releasing them, she's "fluttering," just as a butterfly flutters its wings. Awww!

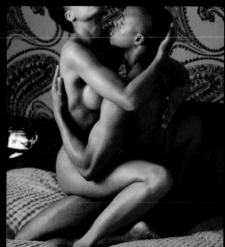

<< STEP THREE

He lifts himself so he's "standing" on his knees, one foot flat on the bed. She stretches out her legs, just as a butterfly does its wings, to move into the final position. Now, unless he spends more time pumping weights than he does pumping her, movement is limited but closely clamped genitals and a unique penetrative angle more than make up for it. The farther she leans back, the greater the pressure. His raised knee makes him more grounded than it seems. If she *gently* moves her body a fraction this way and that, you'll both find a natural balance point.

twining

He might be on top, but winding a leg around his thigh puts her in command of the action for a soul-to-soul sexual smooch.

How to do it

The small, but spiritually significant variation on the standard face-to-face position makes a big difference. She places one leg across his thigh to draw him as close as possible—and puts herself in the power position because she can now use pressure to guide the depth, rhythm, and pace of penetration. Up the difficulty level by doing this position standing up, where it magically transforms into The Vine (see page 132).

Why you'd want to

It's usually a good idea if she's in control because sex tends to be more intimate and last longer. Trade traditional thrusting for circular grinding, moving your pelvises in Elvis-like gyrations.

Hot hint

To alter the depth of penetration, she can move her leg higher or lower; if she turns on her side, it turns into "sexy scissors" for an even tighter fit. For added pleasure, lean forward to allow your nipples to rub against each other or try a *Kama Sutra* style scratch on the back.

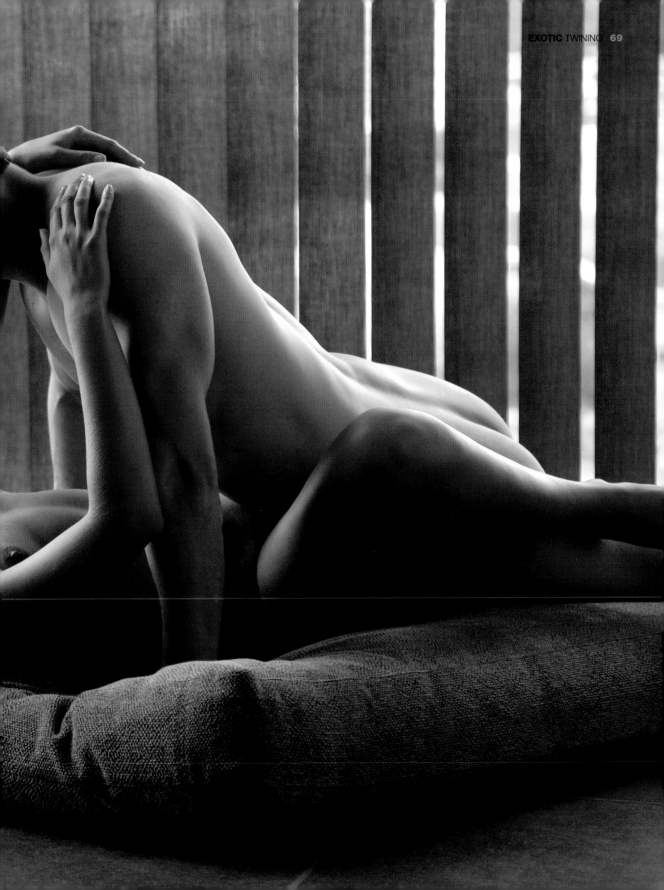

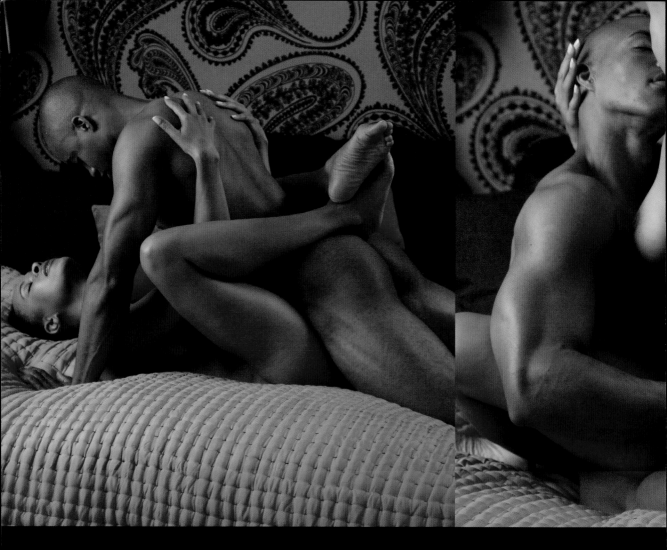

Sex with a secret purpose

DESIGNED TO DO MORE THAN JUST PROVIDE YOU BOTH WITH A PHYSICAL SEX FIX, THESE QUIRKY POSITIONS HAVE SOME HIDDEN BENEFITS...

THE CRANE

Start in the missionary position, him supporting his weight on his hands. She wraps her legs around his waist, crossing her ankles at the small of his back. He climbs "up" her body so he's riding her so high, her pelvis rolls back to put his penis and her vagina in perfect alignment. He then stays completely still as she rolls her hips in small circles, first one way, then the other. The purpose of this is to "heal" and stimulate her sexual organs. Not feeling sexually sick? Try it anyway—it feels fab!

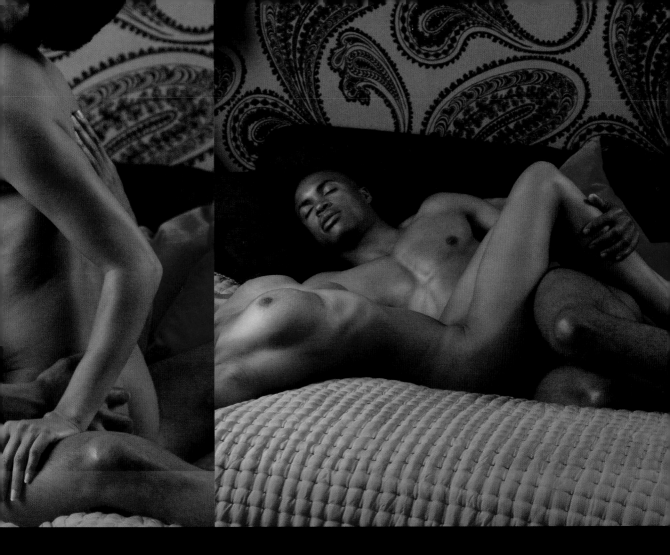

NAKED NUZZLE

There's so much available to nuzzle and nibble in this pose, it's easy to see why it's often a favorite. Penetration is deep and straight forward. All he has to do is push her bottom toward him. If you can drag yourselves away from devouring each other's flesh, lock eyes. Spiritual sex devotees are crazy about seated postures where the couple gaze into each other's eyes for seeming unending periods. And as the eyes are hypnotic windows to the soul, try some erotic eye gazing to read each other's innermost sexual desires.

TAKE A BREAK

This handy little number is designed to be used as a "breather" position, slipped in between more dextrous and demanding ones. You're even allowed to have a little nap if you want (which is sort of in the cards if he's already had an orgasm, has his head on a comfy pillow, and is being flooded by Mother Nature's sleepy post-orgasm hormones!). In theory, his penis would stay inside her as you both sleep. In reality, it will sneak out to snuggle up against his thigh and join you!

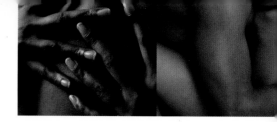

muscle up!

PRACTICE ALL YOU LIKE, BUT YOU AREN'T GOING TO COME CLOSE (OR AT ALL) IF YOU DON'T GET A FIRM GRIP ON YOURSELF. LIKE, LITERALLY. HERE'S ALL YOU NEED TO KNOW ABOUT THE SECRET YONI AND LINGHAM STRENGTHENERS THAT REALLY DO MAKE *ALL* THE DIFFERENCE.

Congratulations if you've resisted skipping straight to the positions and have dutifully read this book in order (you're due for a spanking if you didn't—or better still do it to each other). Now you're ready to shift things up a level or two. You'll both require a reasonable level of physical fitness to master spiritual sex, but I'm actually not just talking limb flexibility or stamina: you need to be skilled at muscle control. We talk a lot about pelvic muscle control for women, but it was the Chinese, more than 3,000 years ago, who first acknowledged that men can achieve multiple orgasms by delaying and/or withholding ejaculation via control of their PC (pubococcygeal) muscle. Kinsey (the famous sexologist) reported a similar discovery in the 1940s, but the concept of multiple orgasms for men never really caught on, probably because it requires holding off. Most men remain resolutely fixed on doing the opposite: getting their rocks off. But, if you want a truly brilliant bam-chicka-wow-wow good time that results in your girlfriend looking at you with limpid, liquid eyes and saying, "You're the best I've ever had," this could provide it.

It's not just the *Kama Sutra* or *The Perfumed Garden* that sing the praises of doing regular pelvic floor workouts. Any sex writer worth their stuff mentions them. But just as owning a huge library of books won't make you well read, simply thinking, "I must do those kegel things" doesn't have the same effect as actually doing them! Your PC muscles form a triangular shape, which stretches from the penis to the anus in men and from the front of the vulva to the anus in women. The benefits of both men and women doing regular PC "pull-ups" are immense (including stopping little spurts of pee coming out every time a new mom has a belly laugh after childbirth.) The fitter and more toned this muscle, the greater the sensation for both of you. The vagina grips the penis nice and tightly, making it better for him *and* intensifying orgasms for her. The exercises also increase arousal because they improve the blood flow to the pelvic area, upping lubrication. So even if you don't achieve the jackpot of multiple orgasms for both of you, regular workouts pay off *big time*.

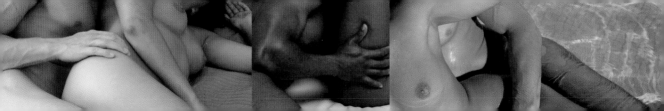

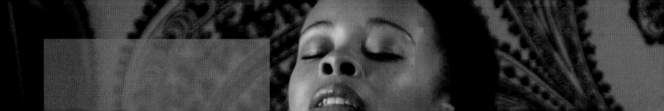

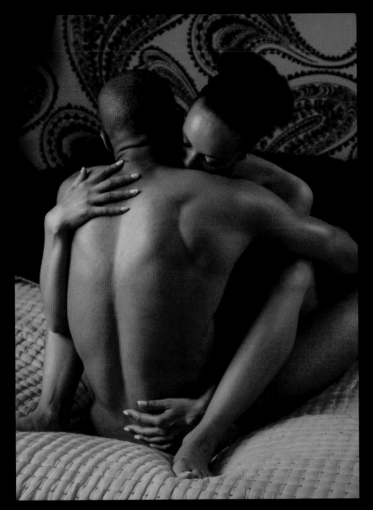

<< STEP ONE

Sit opposite each other, with her legs over his thighs, and embrace. Don't start any funny stuff just yet— you're simply settling into some good old-fashioned necking as you both arouse each other fully in preparation for a good old-fashioned screwing.

STEP TWO

He lifts his legs up until they rest on her shoulders and now penetrates. She pulls him close to her by holding onto his calves and waits for a few moments before pushing herself forward into a wonderfully dominant role.

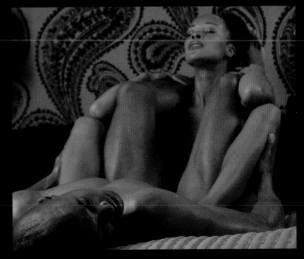

<< STEP THREE

She's now in the "male" position, while he gives in to her wickedly wanton ways and becomes vulnerable. Still struggling to figure out how penetration happens? Well, I struggled with this one (or my boyfriend did anyway). My (boastful) best friend, however, managed it no problems with hers (you can guess what that means!), but penetration isn't always the object with spiritualists more concerned with where the mind and imagination are travelling than your bits.

11

TOP POSITION

mare's position

She jumps on top of him for the ride of his life, literally milking each moment of this erotic roller coaster.

How to do it

Strictly speaking, this is more a technique than an actual position. Unlike the "elephant" (see page 40), it's not inspired by a hot, animal, horsey romp, but refers instead to her "looking after him" by using her pelvic floor muscles to pump his penis to orgasm. The "mare" reference refers to feminine energy and maternal instinct—a girlpower grip!

Why you'd want to

Facing away from him, she places her bod in a fab fondling position. She can put on a frisky floor show by touching her own breasts and clitoris or he can easily reach around to do it himself.

Cheat by...

Unless she's faithfully followed the kegel workout plan (see page 72), it's impossible to cheat with this one. If your internal muscles aren't toned enough to pump and flutter your way to his heart, make up for it with enthusiasm. Thrust away as energetically as you can!

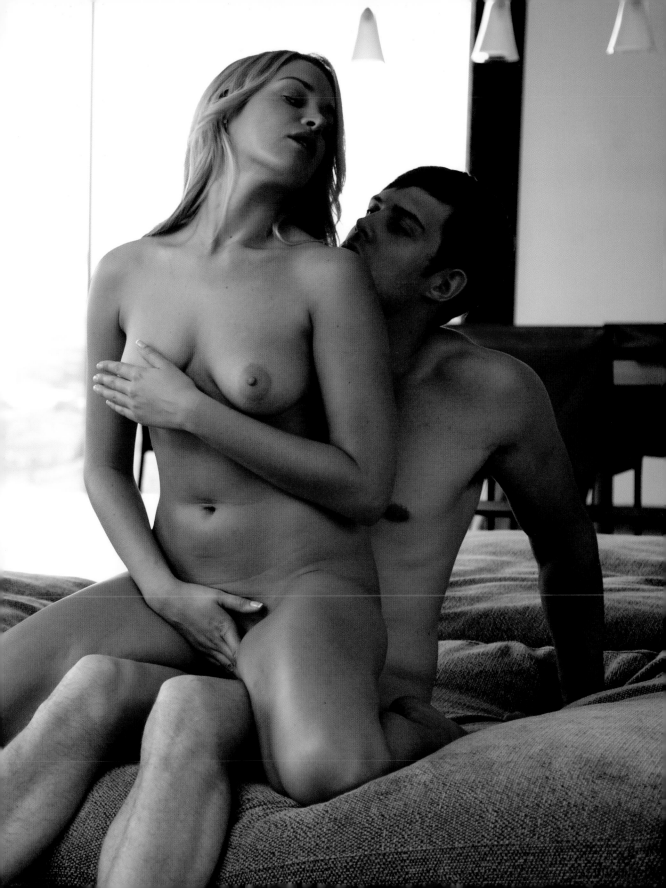

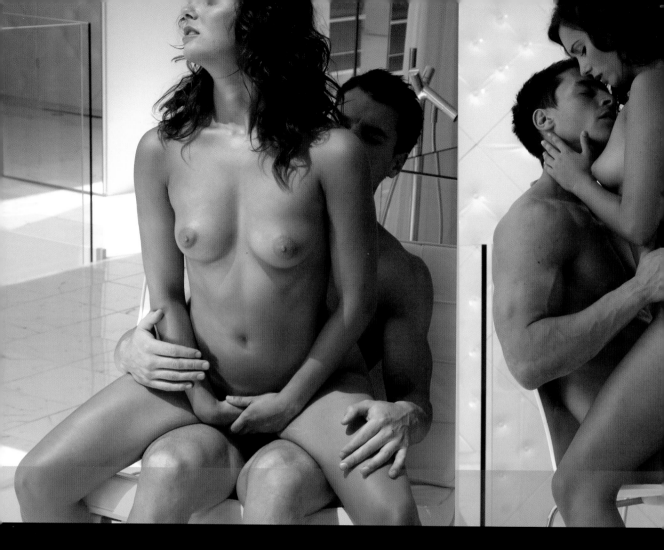

Tender, teasing, and erotic

"COME AND SIT ON MY LAP" JUST TOOK ON A WHOLE NEW MEANING. HOW TO TURN A ROMANTIC CUDDLE INTO A FULL-ON FLESHFEST.

LAPDANCE

This works on a (very stable) chair (minus arms) or on a step—all you need is for him to be able to sit down in the usual way, with her on his lap and your feet flat on the floor. She then lifts herself up and down to rock on his penis. There are obvious advantages to this: first, it can naturally morph from what began as an affectionate moment. Secondly, it's ridiculously easy for her or him to reach down or around to stimulate her clitoris. Meanwhile, she makes like a lapdancer, adding in many a wanton wiggle

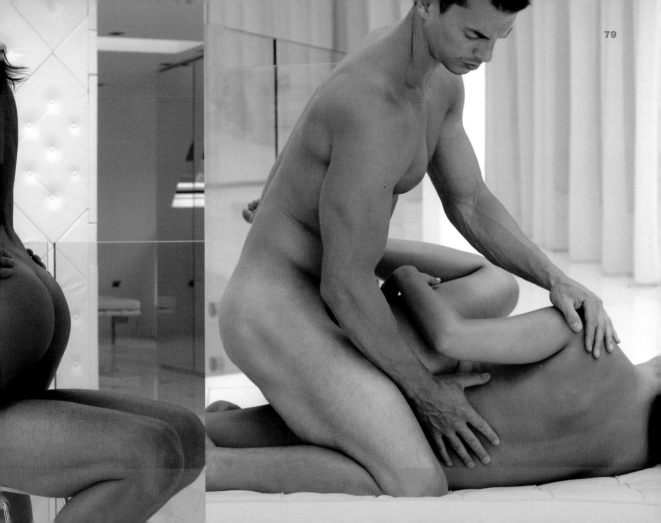

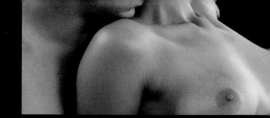

fancy new ways to push

A NEW THRUSTING STYLE CAN TRANSFORM TRIED-AND-TIRED SEX INTO A FRESH, FEISTY PASSIONATE ENCOUNTER WITH ONE TWIST OF A HIP. WANT INTERCOURSE TO BECOME HER NEW FAVORITE THING TO DO IN BED? YOU'VE COME TO THE RIGHT PLACE...

If there's one area where most men are lazy with a capital "L," it's with their thrusting technique. And if you were to film a standard sex session with most couples in the world, 95 percent of men would be thrusting in the conventional way: in-out-in-out (yawn) in-out. Same speed, same depth, same hip motion, same darn everything. I mean, come on guys, is it any wonder lots of women rate intercourse as the least interesting part of sex?

There are 10 different thrusting techniques to choose from, **but don't attempt to accomplish all of the techniques in one session**—we want you to look

TOP THRUSTING TECHNIQUES

Churning He grasps his penis at the base and moves it in circles inside the vagina. Another variation that scores mega brownie points: he holds his penis and she lies back with legs apart while he rubs and flicks the (oh-so-soft) head of his penis over her clitoris until she's close to orgasm. At the last minute, he penetrates and, still holding his penis, "churns" it in circles.

Double-edged sword He strikes sharply downward into the vagina. This is the opposite to modern thinking which has brainwashed both of you to always aim for the front vaginal wall (the bit under the belly)—the location of the G-spot. This is a totally different sensation and, remember, the *Kama Sutra* isn't orgasm focused so has different aims.

Rubbing She raises her hips by putting a pillow under her bottom, he thrusts in a rising (upward) motion. Lots of sex experts (me included) find a multitude of problems solved by putting pillows under bottoms, arms, heads, legs, and various other body parts. It makes everything more accessible and comfortable and alters angles with interesting results.

Pressing The original text says he should press his penis "excitedly" into her womb and hold it there. At first, this seems like a contradiction in terms. Like, if he's super-excited, the last thing on his mind is holding still… unless of course, you're trying to decrease the level of excitement and delay ejaculation. Clever old Vatsyayana—this is exactly when he suggests you use it!

Buffeting He pulls out completely and then penetrates again with a fast, hard stroke. Some women (like me) wince rather than melt at the thought of this. If you've got a sensitive cervix that likes to know what's coming (ahem) and he's rather well endowed, unexpected, deep penetration means pain rather than pleasure. Gingerly test this one out if either of you aren't overly enthusiastic for deep penetration.

Boar's blow He puts continuous pressure on one side of the vagina. One side of the clitoris is often more sensitive, so it could be the case here, too.

Bull's blow He thrusts wildly in all directions like a bull tossing his horns. It should go without saying that attempting this one too early on could mean the whole thing is over before she can say, "That feels grea…" Also not a great one for first-time sex: you risk looking like an overly enthusiastic loon.

Sporting of a sparrow He makes rapid, shallow in and out strokes. If he's close to climax and desperately focusing on an image of his aesthetically challenged mother-in-law in big, gray pants, this isn't the time to try this one. Save it for when he's more in control or… oops, see what I mean?

Sparrow's play He quivers inside her vagina, usually just before orgasm. No need to practice this one really, it just happens of it's own accord. Often right after the previous technique.

The jewel case He gives an involuntary shudder inside her, such as a man makes at orgasm. Ditto.

Moving forward or Natural He gives a gentle stroke forward, which may be varied in depth and speed. Sound familiar? Well that'll be because it's what you do normally (and please God tell me your depth and speed does actually vary a teensy bit!) This is a such a no-brainer, it actually comes without instruction in the original text.

Piercing She lies on her back and keeps her pelvis low (don't raise your hips). He then lies high up on her body (CAT—Coital Alignment Technique—disciples will be familiar with this) and penetrates. The angle of penetration is crucial here. You're not entering at right angles—the usual position—instead the penis is *parallel* to the vulva, so when he moves in and out, it pulls on and stimulates the clitoral area.

Love's tailor He inserts just the head of his penis and makes several small in and out tiny thrusts (aka "sporting of a sparrow"—see above). Then, suddenly, in a single stroke, he thrusts the whole of the penis into her. The idea, of course, is to accomplish several sets of these but don't be surprised if you don't manage to keep it going.

twist and moan

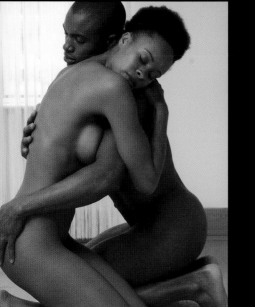

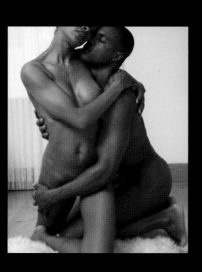

<< **STEP TWO**

He pretty much stays in the same position, while she begins a turn. Putting her left leg over his thighs, he winds an arm around her hips. Pause at this point for him to use his fingers on her clitoris.

^
^ **STEP ONE**

This part's easy: you're both kneeling on the floor, facing each other and taking a moment to simply hug.

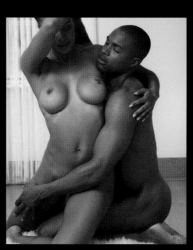

<< **STEP THREE**

Continuing her twirl, she's now put her breasts in prime position to be thrust into his eagerly awaiting mouth. Again, stop for a deep, long kiss and to play with what's laid out in front of you.

<< **STEP FIVE**

Once she's completed her turn, you've both moved into a traditional rear-entry position with him penetrating from behind. In the interests of comfort, it's easier for her to now pull herself up to lean over (and rest!) on a bed or sofa while he kneels behind. Then, let the thrusting begin! After all that pausing, teasing, and acrobatic foreplay you're forgiven if you simply let loose at this point!

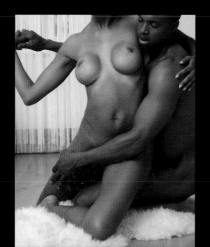

<< **STEP FOUR**

How's her back flexibility? You're about to find out as she twists her spine, pulling her vulva close to his penis and putting herself in a position to allow him to penetrate.

erotic

exotic

exhilarating

exhibitionist

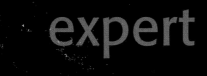
expert

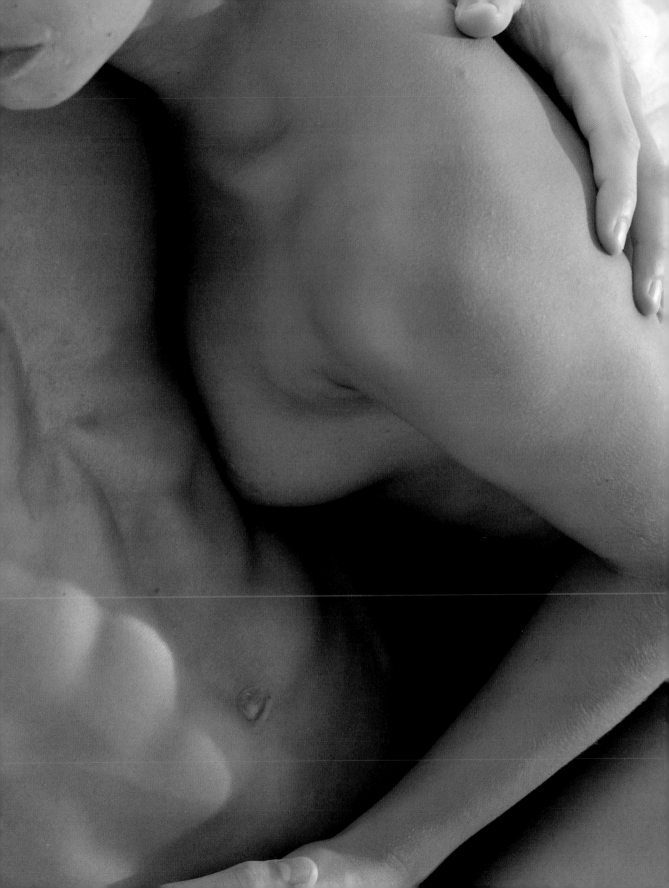

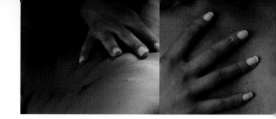

get a grip

HIS HAND AND PENIS ALREADY HAVE A VERY CLOSE RELATIONSHIP, WHICH IS WHY THEY SAY YOU CAN NEVER GIVE A MAN A HAND-JOB BETTER THAN HE CAN GIVE HIMSELF. UNLESS, OF COURSE, IT'S THE TYPE HE COULDN'T POSSIBLY DO SOLO...

The *Kama Sutra* is devoted to the pursuit of pleasure and both Tantra and Taoism place a heavy emphasis on slow, prolonged foreplay. You're encouraged to treat each sexual act in isolation, not as something that gets you one step closer to intercourse. Using your hand to take him right through to orgasm, rather than as a prelude to other things, is something women tend to do at the start of a relationship—particularly during the "let's wait before having full sex" part. Fear of being thought "easy" might stop us proceeding to the penetration stage, but refusing to lend him a helping hand in the meantime seems impolite, if not downright rude. Hence why a hand-job—often mutual—is usually the first sexual act a couple experience. Trouble is, once oral sex and intercourse elbow their way into the bedroom, it tends to get tossed into the "last resort" basket—only to be used if nothing else seems to be getting him there. Spiritual sex devotees say *bull crap* to that! Well, they probably wouldn't say *bull crap*, but they would throw their hands up in horror at today's waste of a sexual act that can be a star attraction in itself. If the only time you wrap your fingers around his penis is during oral sex, he's losing out.

Once oral sex and intercourse elbow their way into the bedroom, hand-jobs tend to get tossed into the "last resort" basket. If the only time you wrap your fingers around his penis is during oral sex, he's losing out.

He's also losing out if you use the same hand technique every single time. Need a few new tricks to freshen up a tired repertoire? Don't just try some of the techniques, give all of them a go! Every single one works *much* better with lube, by the way. So squeeze some onto your hands, and rub them together to warm it up before working some magic. You'll also need to adjust the techniques depending on whether he's circumcised or uncircumcised. If he's "uncut," he'll be a lot more

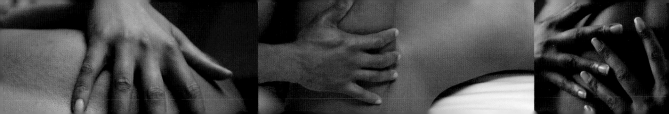

THE TECHNIQUES

Blow-up doll

In this technique, you're imitating the action of a

completely different than the more usual "sliding hand" methods, combining it with a more conventional movement works great.

The corkscrew
Hold the base of the penis with one hand wrapped around it and put your other hand on top in the same position, but holding on to the other side. Start at the bottom and slide to the top, moving your hands in different directions as you wind toward the head. When you get to the head, use the palm of one hand to caress the entire surface then slide your hands back down again to the starting position (it only feels good if you work upward).

Up, up and away
Open your hand so your thumb and fingers are separated to make an L-shaped space, then slide

your hand underneath his testicles until they rest in the space. Push up so you're lifting the testicles slightly, then with your palm down separate the first two fingers of your other hand to make a V and slide his penis between them, working upward from the testicles to the head and tilting your hand so the flat of your hand brushes up against the shaft. Don't just slide up the middle, try sliding up the sides as well, always moving directly upward in a straight line.

Boy scout
Pretend you're a boy scout trying to start a fire by rolling a stick between your hands. Hold the palms of your hands straight, facing either side of his penis and using the rolling/rubbing motion, start at the bottom and slide upward, then down again, keeping a consistent rhythm. Start slowly, then build pressure and speed when he approaches climax.

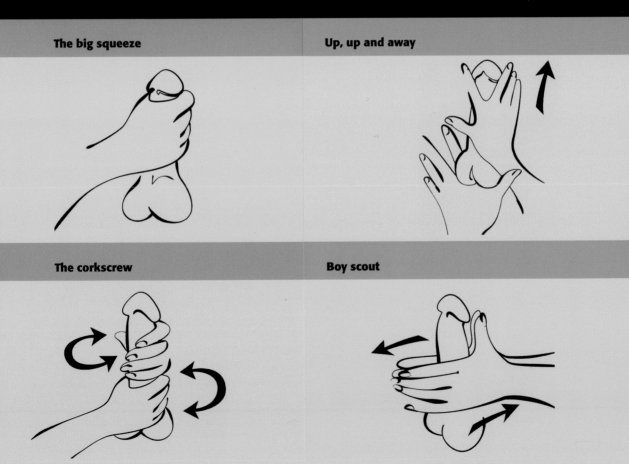

The big squeeze

Up, up and away

The corkscrew

Boy scout

PLAYING WITH OTHER PARTS

If you thought Vatsyayana was dismissive about oral sex, try finding some useful hints about anal play in the *Kama Sutra*. It's barely mentioned, and when it is, airily dismissed as something "some people in southern parts of the country" do. I have no idea what type of people lived in the southern parts back then but I'm guessing they weren't the sort Vatsyayana wanted to invite down to the pub for a beer. Tantrics aren't huge fans either, believing anal intercourse caused a reversal in the natural upward flow of energy in our body.

Listen, I totally understand that anal sex isn't everyone's idea of a fantastic time given the *ouch!* factor. But penises are one thing, fingers and tongues quite another. Approached in the right way, anal play can add a dynamic dimension to conventional sex—particularly hand-jobs. And despite being initially dubious about trying it (it's not just the "Will it hurt?" thing, it's the "If I like it, will it turn me gay?" thing—and no, it won't), most men don't just enjoy the experience, they love it. It's an intense sensation, totally unlike any other, so he might take a few tries to get used to it, but combine anal play with any of the hand techniques here and you're pretty much guaranteeing an orgasm unrivaled by any other.

How to go about it the very first time? First up, don't even think about it if you've got long nails. This only works if they're trimmed below the top of the finger. Secondly, don't attempt it after he's just eaten a big meal—particularly one with lots of cauliflower or baked beans, if you get my drift. The poor guy will be nervous enough, he doesn't need to be worried about passing gas as well! OK, here goes…

HOW TO DO IT

Next time you're fellating or masturbating him, drop to your knees and reach between his legs with one hand to cradle his testicles. Then lick your middle or forefinger (better still: discreetly apply some lubricant) and start playing around the rim of his anus, circling it to begin with, then inserting just the tip. If he pulls your head closer and/or his penis suddenly goes rock hard, you've got permission to take it further. Continuing to suck or manually stimulate him with your hand, gently but firmly start inserting your finger deeper, keeping it curved back toward you. Don't panic if he winces: it can hurt for a moment when you insert your finger but once it's inside, it's actually quite comfortable. Hold your finger still for a moment to let him get used to the feeling, then up the intensity of your hand or blow job and start moving your finger in a "come here" motion, alternating this with sliding it gently in and out and massaging the area. You're now stimulating his prostate gland (the male G-spot) and combined with what your tongue/hand are doing, the end result is usually one hell of a spectacular climax. Don't be surprised if he's absolutely exhausted after it—and a little embarrassed. Our bottoms are intensely private places and associated with not-so-nice things—letting your partner play there can take a bit of getting used to!

RIMMING OR ANALINGUS

This involves licking his anus and/or inserting a stiff tongue inside, thrusting as if it were a penis. It sounds distinctly unappealing for the person doing it but so long as he's emptied his bowels and had a shower, it really isn't. Rimming is a good way to ease him into finger penetration, but also pretty damn exciting on it's own. If you're lying on the bed, get him to turn over saying (with a wicked smile), "Trust me. I won't do anything you don't like." Start by massaging his bottom cheeks, then ask him to lift his bottom. Hold his cheeks open then start licking the part of the testicles you can reach with your tongue, nudging the whole area with your nose. If he starts pushing his bottom higher in the air, he's eager for more. Move your tongue up to his anus and start licking around it, simultaneously reaching underneath him to take a firm hold of his penis. When he's really aroused, use both hands to part his cheeks as wide as possible, stiffen your tongue and thrust it in and out of his anus. It will feel good on his end and the thrill of doing something *so* forbidden can be a turn on for both of you.

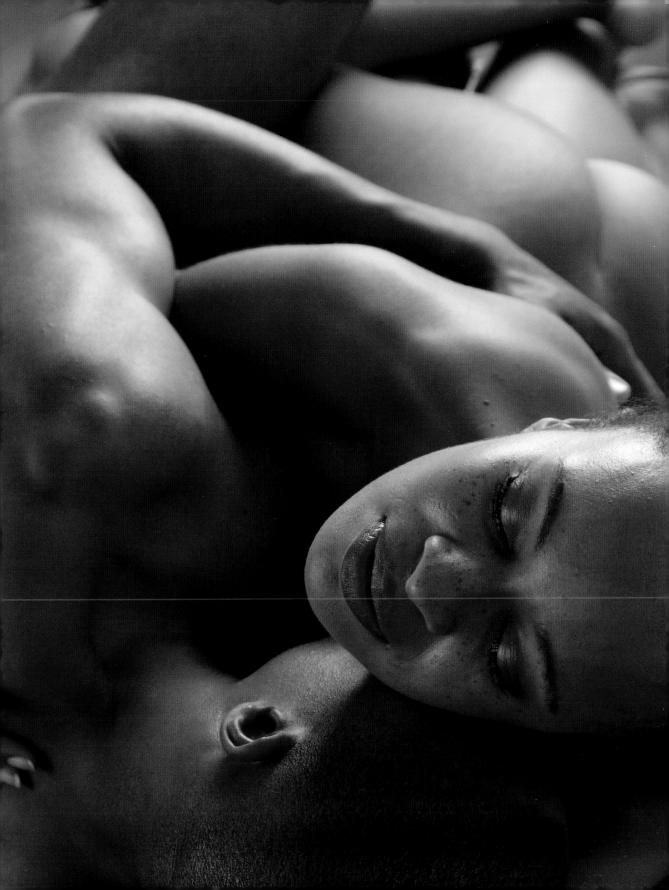

heavenly hand-jobs for her

FEEL LIKE YOU'RE BECOMING A BIT PREDICTABLE IN THE "DOWNSTAIRS HANDS" DEPARTMENT? WANT TO FIND A WAY FOR HER TO ENJOY ORGASMS FROM THREE DIFFERENT HOT SPOTS—SIMULTANEOUSLY? WELL GUYS, JUST SO HAPPENS I MIGHT HAVE THE ANSWERS…

There might not be much detail on how to do it, but rubbing a woman's "yoni" with your hands and fingers until it becomes "soft," gets a definite thumbs up by the *Kama Sutra*. Most of you know how to give your standard hand-job because getting your hands in her panties during her teens, was as far as she'd let you go. Perfecting it to the point where those fingers developed magical powers—like making her panties disappear—was in your interest. But I'd bet your fingers made—and still make—a beeline for her clitoris during manual masturbation, thinking that's the best way to ensure a satisfied smile rather than sulk once your work is done. Well, you're right in one sense—a clitoral orgasm is the most common she's likely to experience. Ancient Taoists, however, believed there were three "gates" of pleasure on the female body. And here's exactly what to do with each of them…

THE FIRST GATE—THE CLITORIS

The clitoris gets No 1 spot and this is the part you already know lots about (if you don't, why don't you?), so I'm going to go straight into it…

Ditch lying beside her for clitoral stimulation Instead sit behind her, get her to sit between your legs and lie back against your chest, then reach around to find her clitoris. Alternatively, bend her over a table or sofa and kiss her neck as you're fingering her from behind. All provide different clitoral sensations and psychological kicks.

How wet is she? Add lubricant if she's not, to make things nice and slippery, then gently part her lips with your fingers and move into the basic stroke: letting your middle finger run back and forth between the inner lips, gently skimming the clitoris each time.

Vary the strokes Switch to sitting in front of her and now hold two fingers in a V-shape around her clitoris (see right), then let your fingers move into a rocking motion. Press them down, using medium pressure, then pull back, then press down—and repeat in a smooth, continuous motion

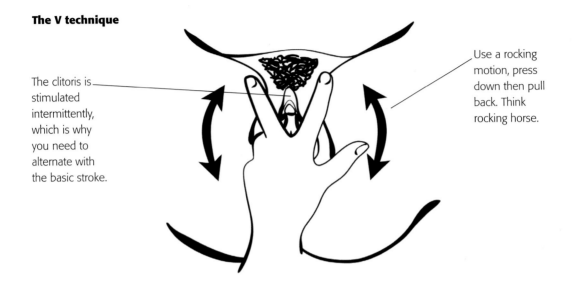

The V technique

The clitoris is stimulated intermittently, which is why you need to alternate with the basic stroke.

Use a rocking motion, press down then pull back. Think rocking horse.

You're doing it right if your elbow is moving back and up. Alternate between this and the basic stroke. **As she nears orgasm** Get her to bear down (push out with her pelvic muscles) to increase the sensation.

THE SECOND GATE—THE G-SPOT:

Okay, this time we're going for something new: "internal ejaculation." What the hell is it? Well, it's a Tao version of the modern world's female ejaculation. Why go there? Well, along with a blissful feeling of "release," her orgasms will be more intense. Which (along with giving her more of them) is the name of the game, right?

The fluid females ejaculate spiritual style is rather romantically called "the nectar of the moon." Unlike our culture which tends to be repulsed rather than delighted by her juices, ancient lovers were positively eager to taste and absorb the "yin" (vaginal) essence because of its many benefits. Today it's the opposite—I get lots of letters from women who are mortified rather than thrilled if they're the ones causing the wet spot, convinced you'll think they've wet themselves!

Here's the challenge: it's your job to make her feel comfortable enough to give this a try indifferent because it's going to be one hell of an experience for both of you if you do pull it off. The orgasm

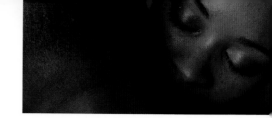

she'll have really will qualify as spiritual because it'll be out of this world and seeing *her* transported to Planet Pleasure provides one hell of a turn on for you, too. (Not to mention earning you the "Best in Bed Boyfriend" award.)

Get this right and the contractions are strong—and addictive. The area doesn't get oversensitive so she's going to want more, and more. And more. Bang goes that Sunday morning golf game.

But before you go diving in (so to speak), take a moment to absorb this crucial piece of advice: the trick to her ejaculating is to encourage her to fight the urge to stop stimulation when the pressure builds to a peak. The first time I had an orgasm, I was utterly convinced I'd see a puddle of pee when I looked down! I didn't (you'll be happy to know) but until you get used to it, the feeling of ejaculatory orgasm can be quite frightening. In order to let it happen, she must allow herself to lose control—and that's something which lots of women find difficult. So before you move on to the physical stuff, make sure her head's in the right place. You can do this by making her feel loved, secure, sexually adored, and by her knowing you won't ever judge her. Reassure her that the feeling of orgasm is simply the release of all the blood that has pumped to her genitals, back into the bloodstream. That's not so scary, is it? Get her to repeat after you: "The only thing that can happen if I let go, is pleasure!"

One other thing, if she doesn't ejaculate (like ever) don't feel like you've failed. Ejaculation is still a hotly contended issue today with some dismissing it entirely, others embracing it, and others saying only certain women can do it. Rest assured though, an orgasm is pretty much guaranteed even if ejaculation isn't. Nothing to lose, everything to gain… Even if you're not convinced there's a specific G-spot, front vaginal wall stimulation is by far the most common way that women ejaculate. The front wall is the side closest to her tummy, which means you're curving your finger/s up and around, rather than simply inserting them. It's not only an awkward position, you have to have damn long fingers to hit it—one reason why G-spot vibrators are selling like mad, because they're shaped to do the job for you. (It's not cheating to buy and use one of these, by the way!). Yes! To work—try the following techniques:

G-spot orgasms However spectacular they are, these involve getting through a not-so-pleasant period where she's absolutely convinced she's about to pee (it's because you're pressing on the urethra). Get her to pee first, so psychologically she knows there's no urine in her bladder.

Get her to sit between your legs Reach around to touch her—or bend her over something and work from behind.

Insert your finger (or the vibrator) Use lube if she needs it, then make a "pulling" motion (like you're beckoning someone over). Use your middle finger—it's usually the longest—and use the others to work on her clitoris. You're attempting to find a small, spongy area which feels ridgy and becomes more raised the more it's stimulated.

Start massaging the area Use more pressure than you would on the clitoris, and alternate massage with the "come here" finger motion. Rather than working around the area, like you would the clitoris at the start, keep massaging directly on the spot and keep going. (I don't care if the game has started—consistency is the key.)

Encourage her to breathe slowly and deeply As she feels the pressure build, get her to deliberately *relax* her pelvic floor muscles rather than tensing them.

THE THIRD GATE—THE CERVIX-

The AFE (anterior fornex erotic zone) lies deep inside the vagina—and I mean deep. It's through stimulation of this area—or even the cervix itself—that her third sensational orgasm can be produced. Like the G-spot, you need fingers like ET or a vibrator/dildo to get to it—or she may need to squat or put one leg up on a chair for you to reach it (not the sexiest pose in the world), But wait, there's good news! You can reach the AFE relatively easily during intercourse. (See, your penis is useful after all!) The best positions to try: she lies on her stomach and you lie on top of her; or she jumps on top, leaning back rather than forward. Because lots of women (like me) associate the cervix with pain rather than pleasure, it's the least publicized of all the hot spots. Getting the end of it swabbed during a pap smear isn't exactly fun, neither is having it knocked during intercourse (like, Owwwwwwwwwwwwww!). But even I managed to overcome all this to become an A-spot enthusiast. Be warned though, get this right and the contractions she feels are strong—and addictive. Unlike the clitoris, the area doesn't get overly sensitive after the first climax. Which, of course, means she's going to want more, and more. And more. Bang goes that Sunday morning *golf game.* Because it's easier to stimulate the AFE during intercourse, I'm going to finish up this bit by giving you the promised multitasker. It's designed to—*tada, dada!*—hit all three gates of pleasure at once and add a fourth dimension! (Forgot the anniversary of when you first met? Offer this as make-up-for-it sex and all will be forgiven.)

Get her in position Put her in a position where everything is virtually laid out in front of you—lying over an appropriate height table would work. You need to have easy access to her clitoris, vagina, and anus with both your hands and your mouth. (She's in for some surprise oral sex a bit later!)

Find the AFE Now insert one or two fingers and set sail for the AFE. You're looking for a patch of sensitive skin just above the cervix (yes, that's miles away!) at the innermost point of the vagina. (You can also buy long thin vibrators which are curved up at the end which do the job nicely.) The difference between this and the G-spot? You're not searching the wall of the vagina beneath her belly, but much farther inside.

Finding the G-spot

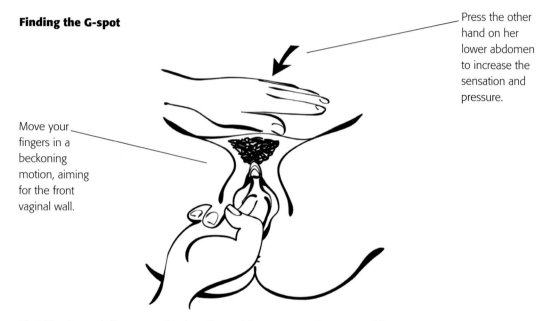

Press the other hand on her lower abdomen to increase the sensation and pressure.

Move your fingers in a beckoning motion, aiming for the front vaginal wall.

Find the G-spot Once you (or the vibrator) has gone as far as possible, start stroking what's hopefully the AFE. After a few minutes of stroking, slide your fingers over the front vaginal wall to massage the G-spot area (or just general area if you can't find a raised bit) using firm pressure (see above).

Alternate between the two Until she's close to orgasm, alternate between the two techniques, then move in to start licking her clitoris—keeping up the stimulation inside with your fingers. The icing on the cake is your final move—inserting one well-oiled finger of your other hand inside her anus. G-spot + AFE + clitoral + anal = the most explosive orgasm experience she's had in her life.

She'll be putty in your hands from now on…

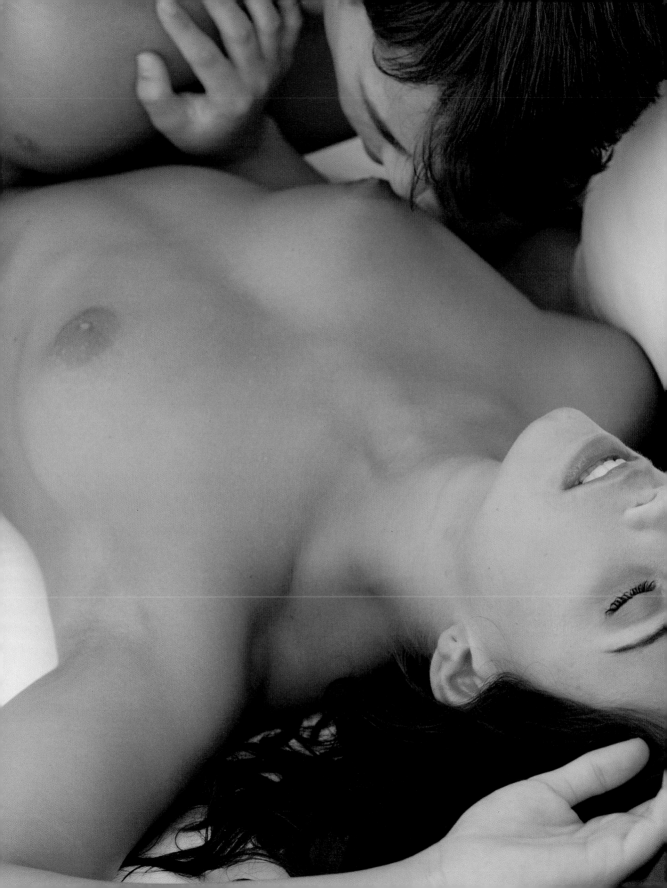

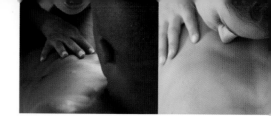

sacred sex sucks

EIGHT NEW WAYS TO ADD FIZZ TO YOUR FELLATIO AND TOP TIPS ON PAYING HIM LIP SERVICE. GIRLS, THERE REALLY IS SUCH A THING AS A BAD BJ!

Given the *Kama Sutra* is the most famous sex book in the world, it comes as quite a shock that oral sex—a cut-your-arm-off-to-get-it pleasure of the 21st century—barely gets a mention. In fact, Vatasyayana is a bit dismissive and uncharacteristically prim on this point. He might suggest eight different ways to perform fellatio, but the only people supposed to practice it were the "third sex" (gay men) or eunuchs on their masters. Only wanton women or serving maids would stoop so low as to give a man oral pleasure (you hussy, you!) Later, he begrudgingly acknowledged that it was okay between partners of the same social standing if their culture permitted it.

Nevertheless, the instructions on giving fellatio is where the *Kama Sutra* slopes off in a wonderfully quirky direction, reminding us rather vividly, that it was written a very, very long time ago when life was very, very different. Like, we might threaten to castrate our boyfriends if they really annoy us—back then they actually did it! Consequently, there aren't too many eunuchs walking around in our society and even if there were, it's unlikely their fate would be to perform the role of a "shampooer." A shampooer was basically a eunuch whose job it was to wash and massage his master, then provide a "happy ending" (if you get my drift). As always, it all had to be done in a particular sequence and fashion. There were eight fellatio techniques and after each one, the eunuch's job was to protest and plead "No more!", waiting for the master to argue and order him to continue before he dutifully wrapped his mouth around… Okay, far too much information, but fascinating in that car crash way all the same. And there are still lessons to be learned from it. What little info is given concentrates on the art of the tease—and never is teasing more excruciatingly, tortuously pleasurable than when performing your partner's favorite sexual activity: the humble blow-job. The second relevant message: variety isn't just the spice of life, adding some unexpected licks and twists to oral sex is the equivalent of adding sparklers to an otherwise boring birthday cake. Want to add fizz to your fellatio? The sequence on page 100 is based on the original eight ways to perform "mouth congress" (fancy for giving him oral sex)—and don't forget to do it in order! As a true *Kama Sutra* student, you'll also stop after each step and wait for him to persuade you before going further. But before you start, here's some other tips you may not know:

STRAIGHT FROM THE HORSE'S MOUTH

I asked a cross section of men to tell me what they considered the secrets of giving great oral sex and all of the usual complaints came up—she doesn't look like she's enjoying it, she thinks she has to suck it like a vacuum cleaner blah, blah, blah. But we know all that stuff already. Here's the more interesting tidbits of what they had to say:

The wetter your mouth, the better The sexiest way to make sure your mouth is nice and slippery. Spit on your fingers (in a ladylike fashion—only joking, don't really think there is one in this instance!), even better put your hand to his mouth so he can do it. Use your hand to hold his penis at the base during oral sex if you're feeling a bit nervous and wobbly. It will stop him from wobbling around as well and give you control.

Not sure how much pressure to use with your hand or mouth? As a general guide, the smaller the penis, the lighter the touch; the bigger he is, the rougher you can be. (Note the words "general guide"—I can't emphasize enough that every bit of sexual instruction is meant as a guide for what *usually applies*. I'm providing a starting point, you then need to vary it to suit him. That's why the word "individual" was invented!) This is because the head of the penis has roughly the same number of nerve endings, regardless of size. If they're spread over a larger area, he's less sensitive.

Concentrate more on the head than the shaft This is because most of the nerve endings are at the head. Don't neglect the shaft though—as your mouth's working on him, use one hand to pump his penis up and down, pulling his foreskin up and over the head if he's uncircumcised, and using a smooth, gliding motion if he's not.

Keep your tongue moving and swirling around to cover as much area as possible, especially when your mouth reaches the head.

Cup his testicles with the other hand and roll gently This is why position is paramount— you need to be in a position where you're balanced, leaving both hands free to work on him. Lying beside him on the bed is the worst position to give great oral sex in; one of the best is kneeling before him as he stands. (If his legs go all wonky when highly aroused, get him to lean against a wall.)

When you want him to orgasm use the side of your hand (thumb pressed between his testicles) and push up firmly between his legs, putting pressure on the perineum (the smooth bit between his anus and testicles). Alternatively, use two fingers to massage the area firmly.

Really, really want him to come? Gently insert a slippery finger into his anus while continuing to fellate him. Leave it still to begin with until he gets used to it, then make a "come here" motion. (I suspect I'm stating the obvious here, but anal play can be a bit of a touchy area. Some men adore it, some men would prefer never to have sex again if it was mandatory. Suggest it, don't force it.)

To swallow easily get in a position where the semen will shoot straight down your throat rather than sit on your tongue in (let's face it) a bit of a congealed, unappealing glob. The trick to swallowing is to do it quickly. If you do, it's there and gone in a second. Let it sit on your tongue for anything longer than a few seconds and there's only way that's disappearing—outward. Discreetly excuse yourself and nip off to spit in the sink or do it in a tissue, handily left by the side of the bed. It's more about letting him ejaculate in your mouth than it is the swallowing anyway. While we're on the subject of swallowing, how he tastes is almost entirely dependent on his diet. If it tastes bitter or pungent, get him to ditch spicy food, beer, cut down on dairy, eat lots of fruit and vegetables and drink lots of water and fresh juices. He's given you a withering stare for suggesting it? Tell him why and he might rethink…

EIGHT NEW WAYS TO EXCITE HIM

Here's the techniques. I've renamed them, but the original *Kama Sutra* name is in brackets.

The warm-up (nominal congress) Put his penis in your mouth and move it around.

Get your teeth into it (biting the sides) Use your hand to hold him still and start nibbling the sides of your penis with your lips. Start with one side, then move down to the other. You're mainly "biting" with your lips, but throw in teensy, gentle nips and see how he responds.

Kiss it better (pressing outside) Did it hurt, diddums? There, there… here you're simply pressing your lips against the head of the penis and kissing it better.

Let the teasing begin (pressing inside) Now put it farther into your mouth then "press" it by tightening your lips. Take it out again, then repeat. By the way, for this technique to be effective, he has to relinquish control once you're doing your stuff. A little bit of tussle is allowed since he's convincing you to continue, but the old push-the-back-of-your-head-down thing will just turn it in back into your average BJ. Does he want something special or what he always gets?

Lip service (kissing) Hold his penis in your hand, then tuck your bottom lip into the corona, the ridge which separates the head from the shaft. Find his frenulum (the stringy bit) and consistently nudge it with your lower lip. By the way, a lot of these movements are subtle: if he's looking distinctly unimpressed, move swiftly on to the next.

Tongue action (rubbing) Go for a bit of tongue action—lick his penis all over, then concentrate on tonguing the opening of the urethra (the little hole at the top which he pees out of), pushing your tongue gently into it.

Suck it and see (sucking a mango fruit) Take him halfway into your mouth, then suck vigorously. I know, I know, sucking is usually considered a schoolgirl error, but after all that teasing, feeling the whole thing enveloped in your warm mouth again is extraordinary. Sucking hard adds to the contrast between playful licking and serious mouth work. This is why the following is called…

The grand finale (swallowing up) "Swallowing" isn't quite what it sounds like because Vatsyayana not only didn't really approve of heterosexual fellatio, he most certainly didn't encourage your partner ejaculating in your mouth. By swallowing, Vatsyayana simply means taking the whole penis into your mouth as if you were trying to swallow it. But since by this stage, he shouldn't just be ready to orgasm, he'll be gagging for it, the likelihood of this happening is about as reliable as knowing you'll have a hangover on Saturday if you agree to a "few drinks" out with the girls after work on Friday night.

The *Kama Sutra*'s instructions on fellatio remind us, rather vividly, that it was written a very, very long time ago when life was very, very different. **We might threaten to castrate our boyfriends if they really annoy us—** back then they actually did it!

The warm-up

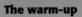

Lip service

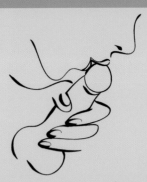

Get your teeth into it

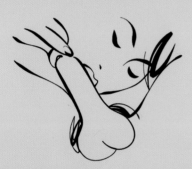

Tongue action

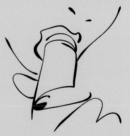

Kiss it better

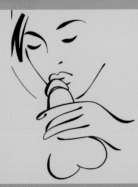

Suck it and see

Let the teasing begin

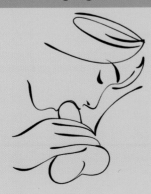

The grand finale

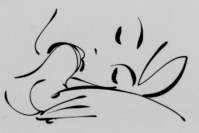

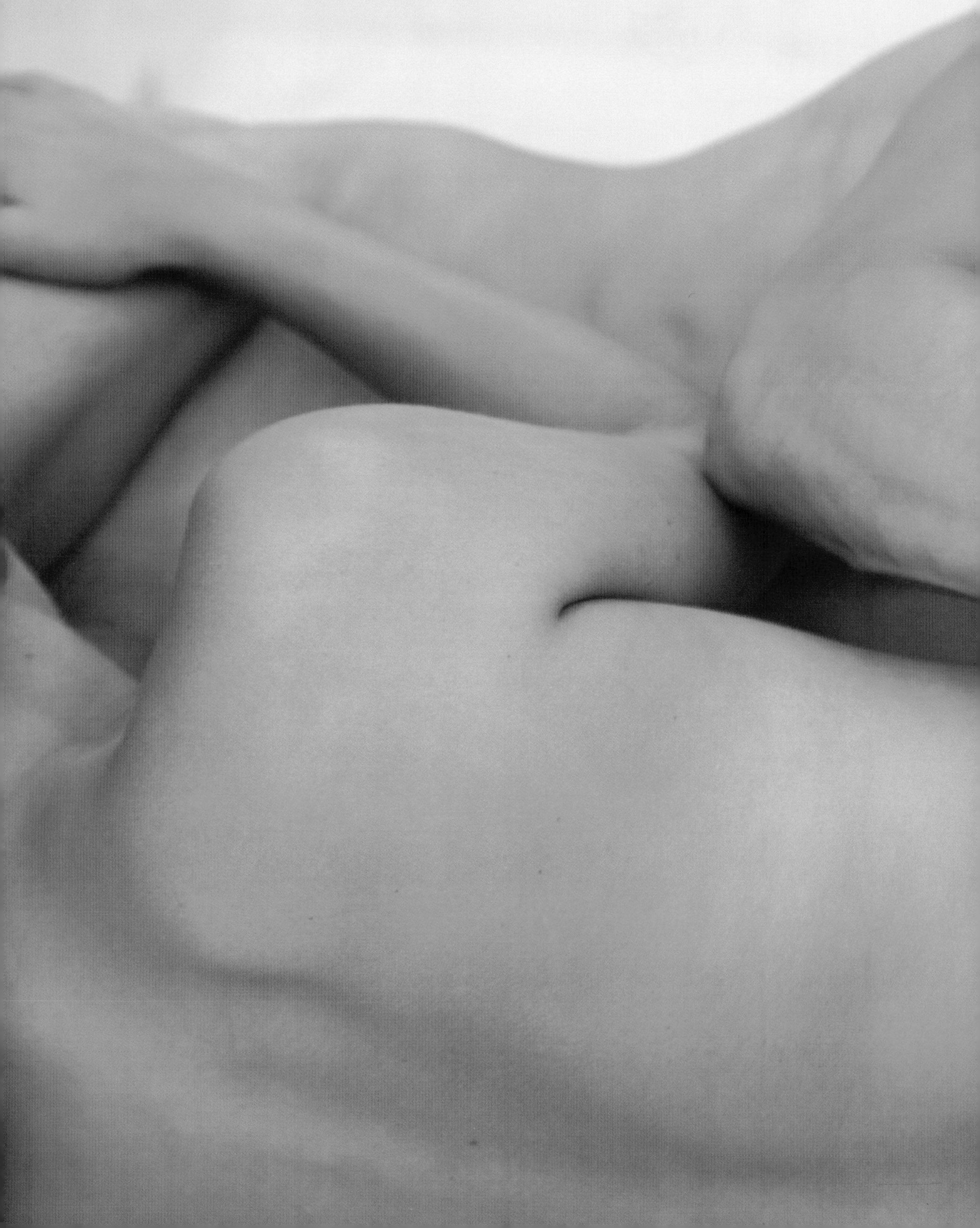

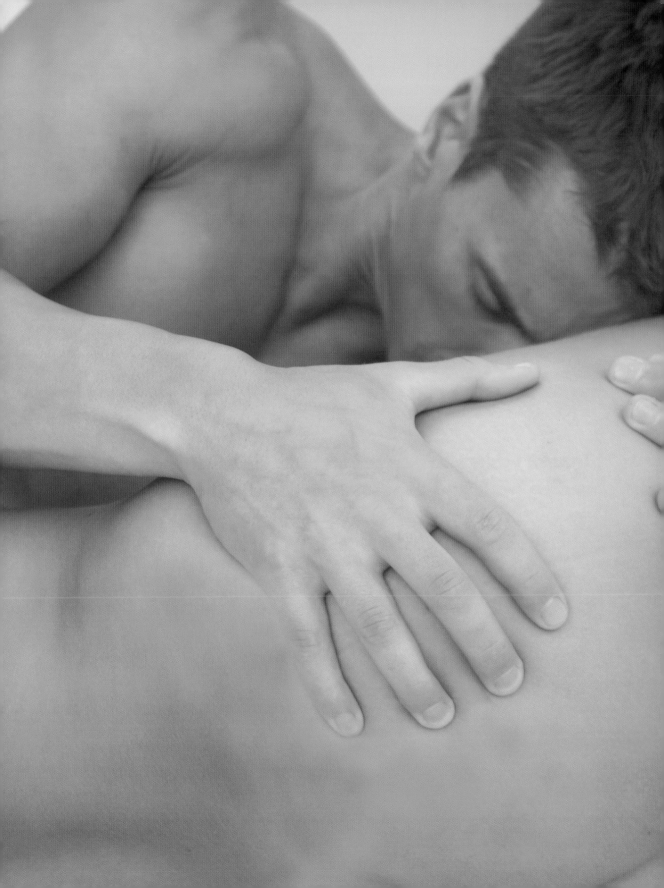

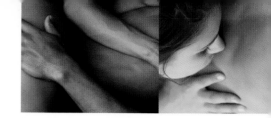

the lowdown on going down

THE *KAMA SUTRA* RATHER NAUGHTILY IGNORES INTIMATE INSTRUCTION ON GIVING HER ORAL PLEASURE. BUT THAT DOESN'T MEAN WE'RE GOING TO! HERE'S HOW TO GIVE CUNNING CUNNILINGUS.

There's fleeting mention of oral sex for him in the *Kama Sutra*—and even less for her! Some say it's because it's biased toward male sexual enjoyment, but I honestly don't believe that. There's way too much emphasis on pleasuring women—long, drawn out methods for seducing her which take weeks or months to lead to so much as a kiss, and strict instructions on how to read the signs her body is ready for sex before a penis so much as waves at her bits. For Vatsyayana to avoid instruction on oral sex simply because it's way too much fun for females, doesn't fit. It's far more likely to be for cultural reasons.

Ignore what you've seen in porn films—they've pulled back and exaggerated the tongue movements so you can see what's going on. In real life, she's unlikely to see anything other than the top of your head.

Interestingly, Tantrics and Taoists don't focus much on it either. So the next logical question is… why am I? Well… hmmmm, let's see. One good reason might be because THIS IS HOW MOST WOMEN HAVE ORGASMS! I'm sorry, did I shout that?

Thing is, even if Vatsyanana didn't wax lyrical about fellatio, he at least threw in eight new tricks for her to try on you, which I've dutifully passed on (see page 100). So if the spiritual meanies won't deliver, I will to make things fair! I asked a selection of men to give her the heads up on giving you head (see page 99), now it's your turn. I'm assuming you know the basics of cunnilingus (if you don't, my other books *Hot Sex* and *supersex* both have good guides), so I've just included the juicy bits (so to speak), but read on for what women believe are the crucial steps to getting it right.

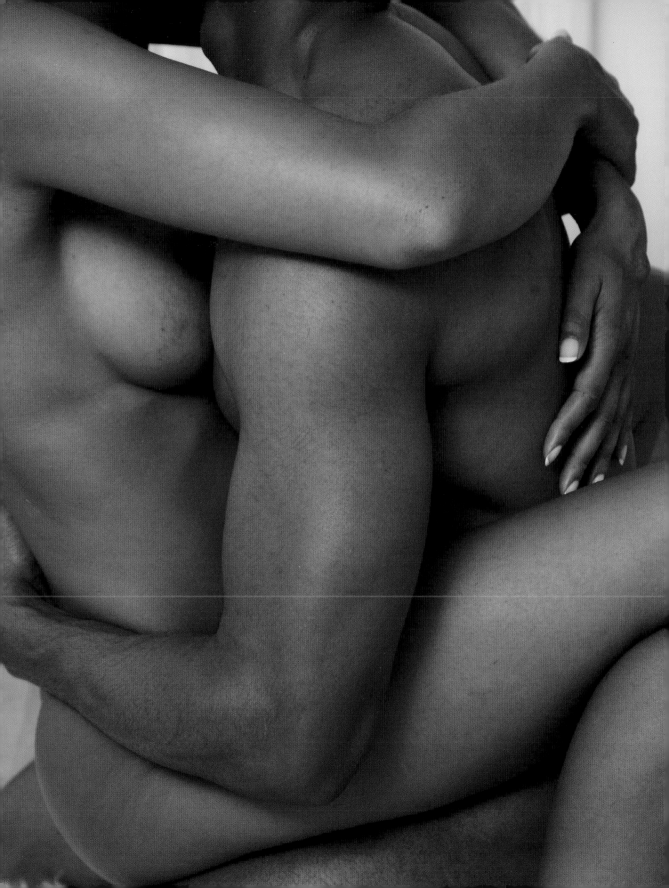

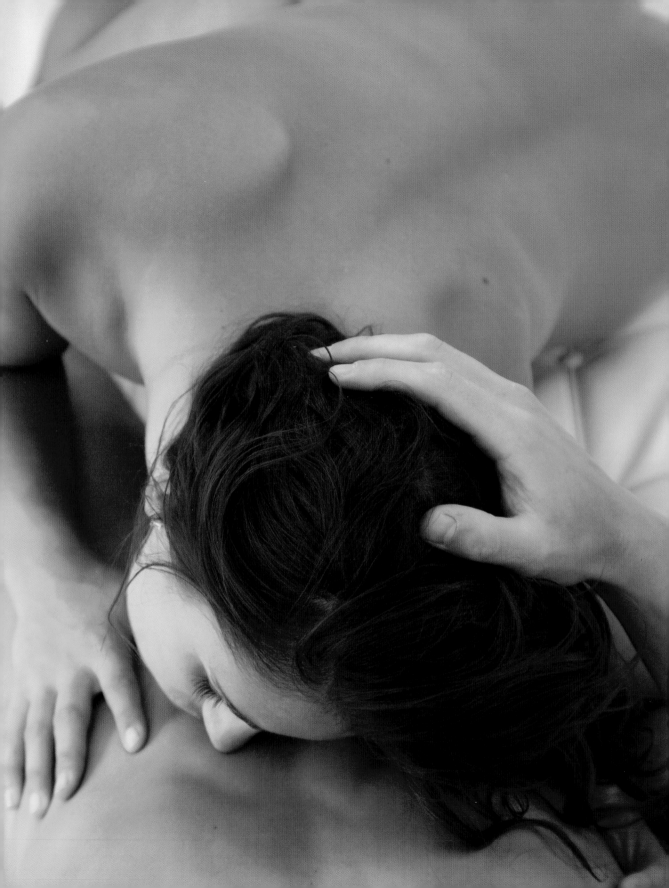

HER TIPS ON WHAT WILL MAKE YOU GREAT

Ignore what you've seen in the porn films— they've pulled back and exaggerated the tongue movements so you can see what's going on. In real life, it's unlikely she'll see anything other than the top of your head squashed between her thighs (and yes, this is the moment she's likely to notice that comb-over you've got going to disguise that bald patch). Flicking with a tensed tip of the tongue can feel great, but the most popular technique is to use the whole flat of your tongue and wiggle it or lick, slowly and consistently in between the inner lips and around and over the clitoris.

Lots of women take up to 20 minutes to orgasm via your tongue You're in there for the long haul honeybunch, so get into a position you're comfortable in. We're already worrying if you're getting bored or your tongue's about to fall off, stressing about a cricked neck isn't going to help either of you. The most comfortable position is probably her straddling your face, hanging on to the wall behind, with a pillow or pillows supporting your neck. If she's a bit too shy, pull her over to the edge of the bed and kneel in front of her. (A kitchen counter also works great—never mind the hygiene issues.)

Read her body language Lots of women are reluctant to tell you what they want and need, so you need to be alert to her body language. Pay attention to any pressure from her hands if she's holding your head. Pulling you closer means tongue me deeper, pushing it away means you're being too rough. Slow everything down, relax the pressure, and simply lick gently. If she's holding you firmly but seems relaxed, you've got it right.

Test techniques, don't just assume she likes it Lots of women are people pleasers and want you to think you're doing a fabulous job, even if they're hating every second of it. Make it abundantly clear you aren't going to be offended and need and want direction from her. While you're getting to know what turns her on, try something for a bit then pull back and ask if she liked it. If you or she find it off-putting to be constantly stopping, try out different tongue movements while making eye contact with her and get her to say "yes" or "no" to each one (even better to be more specific "That was great, but do it a lot gentler" or "Switch between the last one and this one"). Some women, for instance, love their clitoris being sucked. Others (like me) hate it sooooo much, one suck on the clitoris can undo all the good work you've just done for the past 10 minutes. Find out what she likes by putting your lips around the sides of her clitoris, pursing them, and *gently* sucking—then ask her if she enjoyed it.

Sticking your tongue inside her vagina This can be a huge turn-on, but it's unlikely to make her orgasm. You need to combine it with consistent stimulation of the clitoris. While we're on the subject of penetration, be aware that while some women love you inserting your fingers during oral sex, others find it distracting. Tongue movements are subtle and can be outshone by the feeling of penetration which is more aggressive. How do you know what suits her? You know the answer—ask her!

Stop your tongue from getting tired Keep it relaxed rather than tensed, and take little breaks where you move your head rather than your tongue. Or press the flat of it against her clitoris and simply hold it still, letting her move her hips. Make it easier by holding her vaginal lips open and pulling the whole labia up to make her clitoris more visible.

Reach new spots by drawing a figure of eight on her clitoris or write "Jesus, I wish you'd hurry up because my tongue hurts." Anything to ensure you're hitting a part of her you haven't before.

A dry tongue feels like sandpaper, a wet one feels simply marvelous. If you're horribly hungover and dehydrated, keep some water beside you and swig it.

Simultaneously press down on her lower abdomen to arouse the part of the clitoris which isn't visible. (The part you see is just the tip!)

Keep everything super wet A dry tongue feels like sandpaper, a wet one feels simply marvelous. If you're horribly hungover and dehydrated, keep some water beside you and take a few swigs if you need to. It's not ideal but believe me, she'd prefer a brief interruption than a whole session of dry cunnilingus. Alternatively, put your fingers up to her mouth and get her to "spit" on them (but only if she's got a wicked streak).

Think about the direction of how you circle her clitoris It feels quite different clockwise and counterclockwise. Try mixing it up a little—a few twirls one way, a few twirls the other. As a general rule, the smaller the circle you're making with your tongue, the more intense the stimulation; the larger the circle, the less intense. Start off with large circles, making them smaller as you go along.

Avoid desensitization Make sure you don't concentrate on exactly the same spot the entire time—unless of course, she wants you to! If she seems to have been enjoying it but isn't now, even though you're doing exactly the same thing, she's probably been over-stimulated to the point of numbness. Reach new spots by drawing a figure of eight on her clitoris, spell her name—or write "Jesus, I wish you'd hurry up because my tongue hurts." Anything to ensure you're hitting a part of her you haven't before.

Have a good look at her clitoris to see how exposed it is If she's got quite a large clitoris and it's easily exposed from under the clitoral hood (the little hood of flesh which covers it), you need to be gentler with your tongue strokes than if her clitoris is

small and hiding shyly away. If it is, place your lips around it to bring your tongue closer and work more specifically. Pull the flesh of her mons upward to make it more visible or get her to lie back, you kneel at right angles to her and place two fingers on either side of the hood of her clitoris to "pop" it out.

Pace and pressure You may prefer to up the pace and pressure as you approach orgasm, but she may not. A lot of women would rather you continue the same rhythm, which got her close to orgasm in the first place, rather than step it up. Others like you to actually be gentler.

Make noise If you're trying to help tip her over the edge into orgasm, moan to let her know you're as turned on as she is. (A brilliant compliment to say to her afterward: "I almost came when you did, that was such a turn-on.") If she's into penetration, insert a finger/s inside, reach up to play with her breasts, or (again, if she's into it) put your thumb inside her anus.

Throw in some analingus She'll be shy and probably protest the first time around, so take baby steps and work up to a full session. Try pushing her forward over a sofa and ask her to part her legs and push her bottom high in the air as she leans on it. This gives you easy access to her clitoris and anus. Position yourself behind her and start by pushing your tongue forward, so your tongue tip is playing with her clitoris. Even if you don't want to stimulate her anally, the angle and position makes oral sex feel different—and the fact she's exposing herself to you is also a huge turn on. Once she feels comfortable and aroused, start licking around her anus. Is she seems to like that, hold the cheeks of her bottom apart and start pushing a stiff tongue inside her anus, teasing her clitoris with your fingers at the same time

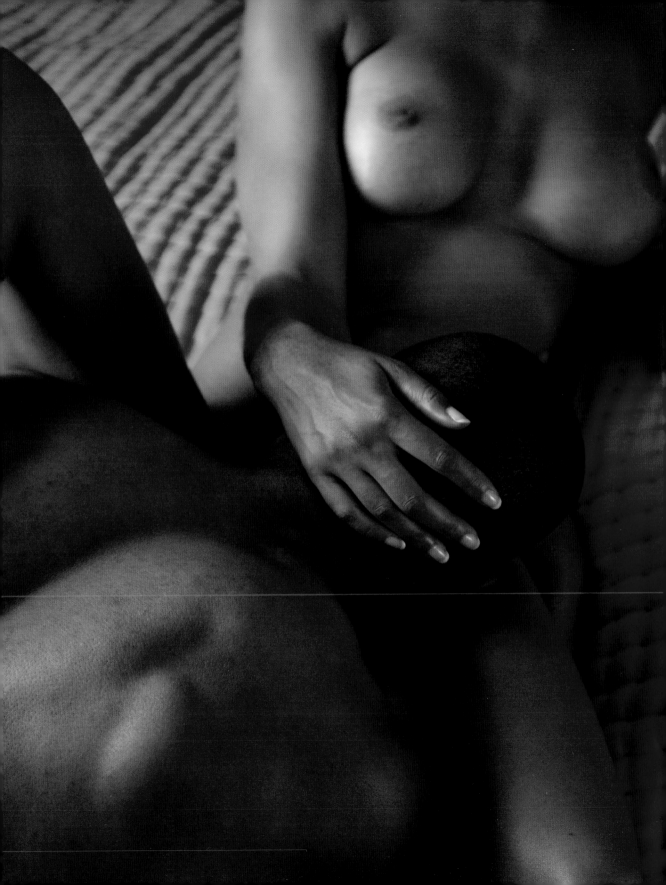

erotic

exotic

exhilarating

exhibitionist

expert

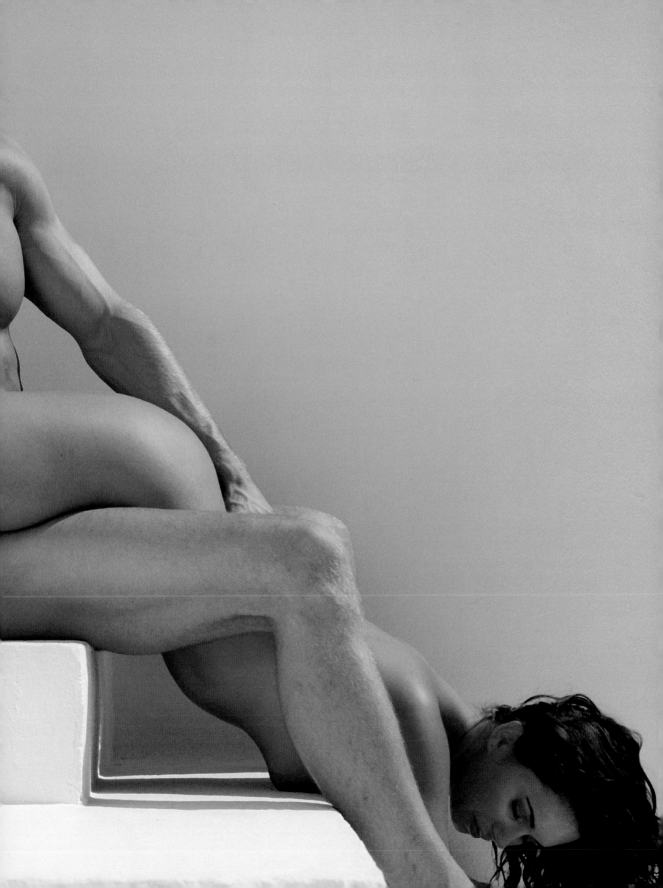

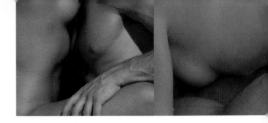

what's your sexual fit?

IS HE A HARE, A BULL, OR A STALLION? FIVE FINGERS OR 10 INCHES? ARE YOU
A DELICATE DOE OR... AN ELEPHANT? INDEED! A LOOK AT (THE DECIDEDLY
ODD) *KAMA SUTRA* TAKE ON GENITAL SIZE—AND HOW YOU CAN SPOT EACH
OTHER AT 20 PACES.

Slightly insecure about the size of your genitals or your looks? I suggest you quickly flip the page or,
if your partner insists on reading out bits, put your hands firmly over your ears and say "Tra-la-la"
until they stop. The way a couple fit together both physically and sexually is taken *very* seriously
by Vatsyayana: compatibility is a central theme of the *Kama Sutra*. To ensure everyone finds their
matching sexual bookend, he kindly divides us into three classes dictated by the length of your
lingam (that's penis to you) and the size of your yoni (her vagina). To be even more helpful, he
then helps you predict what's hidden below by how the person looks. And it ain't pretty. None
of this tiptoeing around, protecting the delicate male ego or a woman who's self-conscious after
giving childbirth by putting things tactfully or observing any form of political correctness. Vatsyayana
cuts straight to the chase. Well-endowed men get to be proud, mane-tossing, studly "stallions";
guys who weren't first in line when God handed out willy genes are called "hares"—mousy, jittery,
fast (and everyone knows while "a stallion" is on every young girl's wish list, hares never are).
And men get it easy. Women with vaginas on the, err… larger side are clumsy, gray, wrinkled old
"elephants," while their small sister is a big-eyed, long-limbed, ultra-feminine "doe."

Girls, hang on to your sense of humor or close any open windows and remove all sharp objects.

If you're already feeling insulted, for God's sake get over it. The male descriptions of what you're
likely to look like are quirky to say the least, the female is so derogatory, they're roll-around-on-the-
floor funny! In his defense, Vatsyayana doesn't deliberately set out to upset—or compliment—us.
He's simply trying to ensure there's true, pure sexual compatibility. Morbidly curious to know which
category you fit into? Get out the tape measure, guys. Girls, hang on to your sense of humor or
close any open windows and remove all sharp objects. The really good news for all of you: it's all
a load of bull. Don't take it personally, I just couldn't resist including it for a laugh!

FOR HIM

Hare Around six fingers or approximately 5 in (13 cm) long. There's no way of putting this delicately, guys: if this is you, you're the smallest—but I bet you have lovely eyes and a terrific personality. (Sorry, wrong to joke at a time like this.)
What you look like: You've got small feet and teensy buttocks, hands, and ears. Your voice is gentle, you've got beautiful and well-spaced teeth, a round face, and you're always smiling. There's nothing offensive about your semen.

Bull Around eight fingers long or approximately 7 in (18 cm). What is there to say? You're Mr. Average.
What you look like: You've got a thick neck, impressive bearing, red palms, an assured air, clear skin, a nice round tummy—and you're always lucky.

Stallion About 12 fingers long or approximately 10 in (25 cm) inches. Alright you smug bastard, you knew you'd win.
What you look like: You've got elongated ears, head, and lips. A thin body, thick hair, long fingers, and heavy thighs. You're a "fast" person and have beautiful nails. (Hah! You thought you were going to be rippling with muscle, didn't you!) Your semen is copious, salty, and "goatlike."

The really good news: Hares swell to stallions on special occasions (just got out of prison/been asked to road test all the contestants on *America's Top Model*).

FOR HER

While he's specific on penis size, Vatsyayana doesn't give measurements for females, simply a vague "width and depth of the vagina." The man is supposed to figure this out himself, based on his penis size and how it fits inside her. All a matter of subjective judgement. (Hands up, if you're a doe then?)

Doe/deer—a small vagina. Deep penetration often hurts, you often need to add lubrication for him to penetrate unless you're massively aroused—and premature ejaculation happens so often, you have no idea it's not the norm.
What you look like: You've got beautiful hair, a thin body, narrow face, golden skin, strong teeth, a low voice, and abundant hair. You don't eat much, your sexual secretions are scented, you never cry out and have a vagina as "cold as the ray of the moon." Think your average supermodel with a low sex drive.

Mare—an average vagina. You've never had any complaints but do have the odd paranoid urge to ask "Am I tight enough?". If you've had a child, you religiously did your kegel exercises (or took the easy way out and asked for "a husband's stitch"). It's only if he has a large penis that penetration is a problem.
What you look like: You have wide, strong nostrils and are slightly knock-kneed with thick thighs and a vagina which is always hot. You've got tender, fat, sweaty arms, regular limbs, a small belly (well that's good) and sexual secretions that smell of meat (not so good). Not surprisingly, given you're walking around smelling like cooked cow, you're often bad-tempered and irritable.

Elephant—large vagina. Blame it on your mother (it can be genetic), your six kids (who's got time for kegels?), or that bottle of vodka you just drank (alcohol doesn't just relax the mind). You're tempted to use the phrase "Is it in yet?" rather often.
What you look like: You're tall with a strong, massive body, long teeth, reddish-colored skin and you have an unpredictable vagina—it's sometimes cold and sometimes hot. You talk a lot and your vaginal secretions smell like (wait for it) elephant sweat. There! And you thought the news would be all bad! (There was a reason for telling you to close all open windows.)

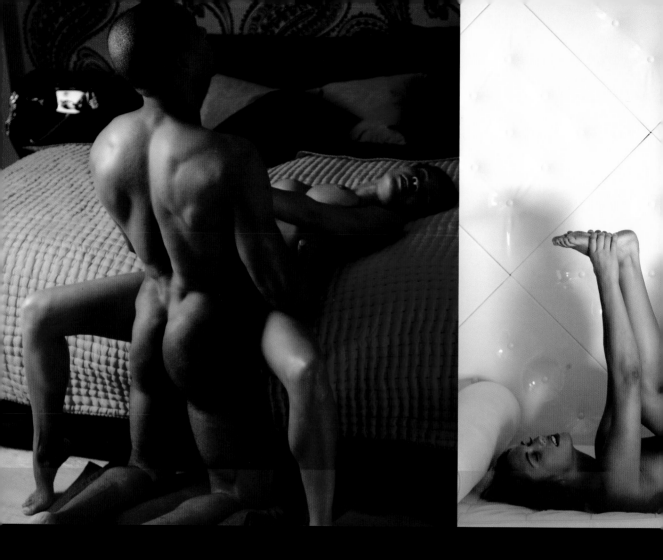

From ordinary to extraordinary

OLD FAVORITES GET A NEW LIFE—AND HE GETS TO SIT DOWN ON THE JOB. LITERALLY. DON'T BE ALARMED, THOUGH—ALL IS NOT QUITE AS IT SEEMS...

THE EDGE

This is inspired by a Tao position, but it's already a favorite for lots of couples because it manages to satisfy two appetites simultaneously: the need for both hot sex and comfort! He kneels on something soft, she positions herself on the edge of the bed and opens her legs *wide* so he can enter her. He takes firm hold of her hips and moves her up and down on his penis. Simple. Damn effective.

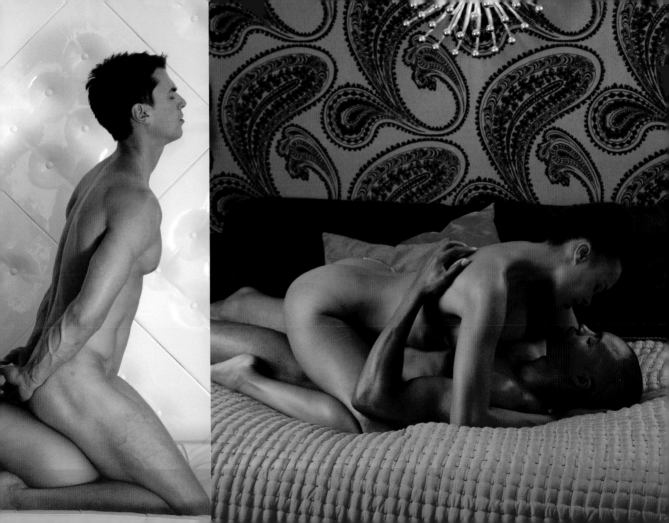

12

TOP POSITION

the cow

A perfect position for spontaneous sex—
and great for feeding those naughty,
anonymous stranger fantasies.

How to do it

She plants her feet wide apart for balance and bends
over until both her hands are flat on the floor. He
enters from behind and holds her by the hips to
enable him to thrust.

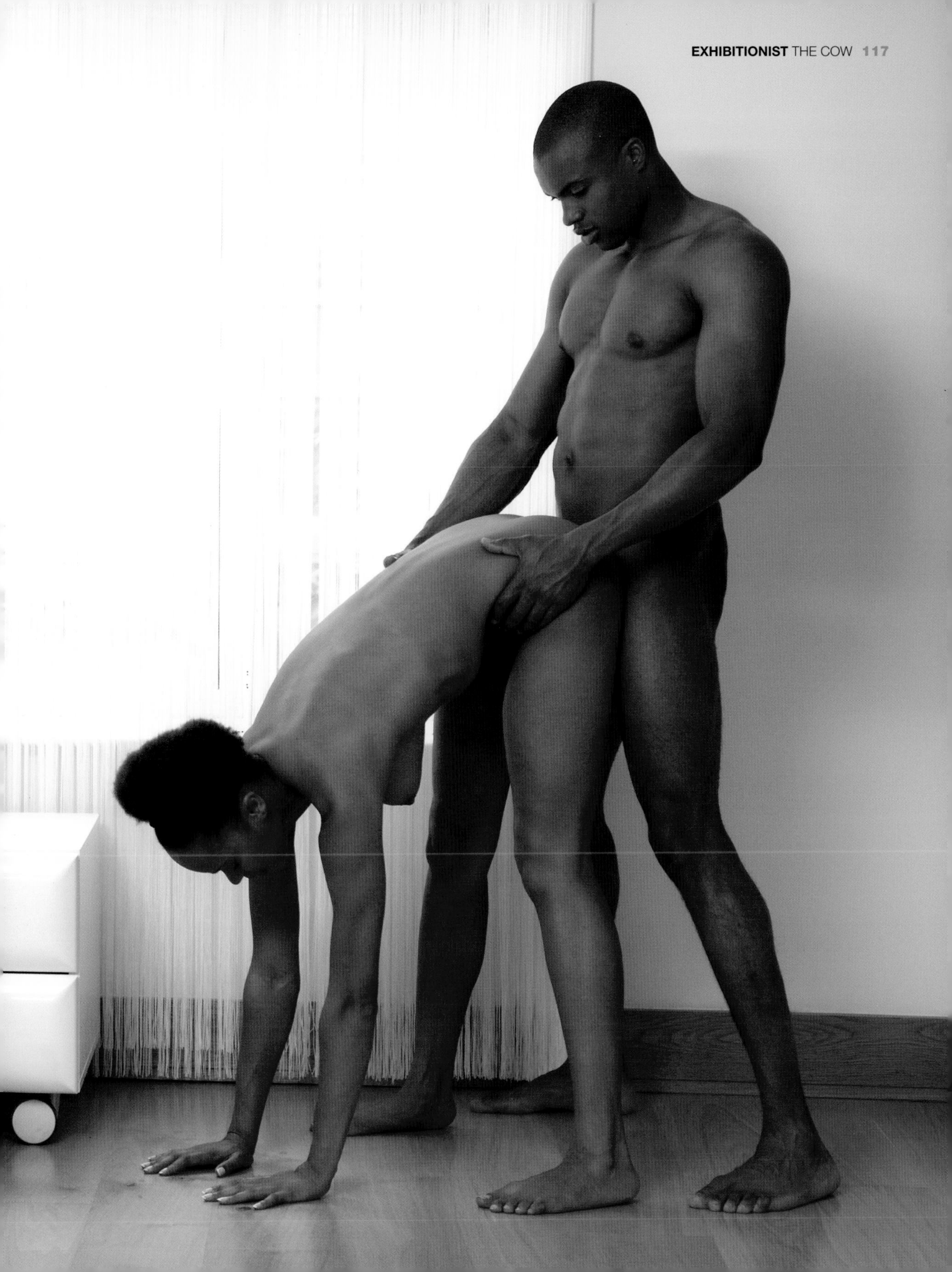

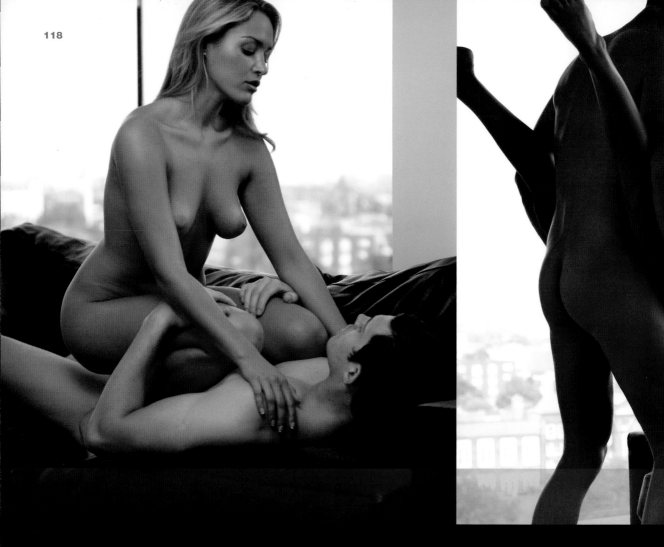

Gym for your genitals

SQUAT, STRETCH… AND THEN RELAX. START OR COMPLETE A HIGH-ENERGY, ASPIRATIONAL SEX SESSION WITH A LOW-STRESS OPTION.

THE WANTON WORKOUT

Instead of sitting astride him with knees and calves supported either side, she squats. It might not be as comfortable, but it's easier to move. Continuing on from the "woman satisfying herself" theme (which we're loving, by the way), the main plus of this is that it's easy for her to rub herself against him, back and forth, providing much-needed friction on the clitoris. Assuming her thighs can take the pace, she's in control of how deep he goes, the type of thrusting used, the angle he penetrates, and how fast and hard he pumps.

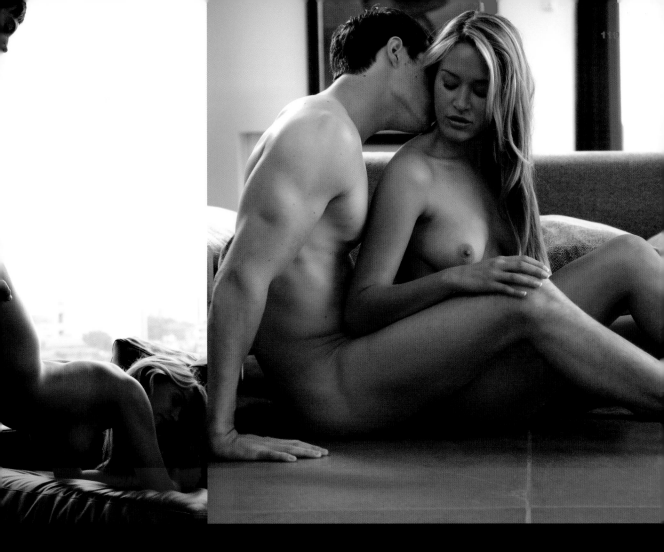

CLASSIC WHEELBARROW

This is the one most new-to-sex men want
to attempt. They've seen pictures of it, and it
not only looks downright he-manish but
achievable. She leans face down on a piece
of furniture that's an appropriate height,
resting her weight on her forearms. He
kneels behind her, penetrates, then stands
(straining every step of the way), pulling her
up with him. She stretches her legs out once
they're in position. It's hard work, so save
it for those just-about-to rather than I-could-
go-on-forever occasions.

LOVING LEAN

This position can be the prelude to a sex
session… or a romantic finale. He sits
and she settles between his legs, facing
away from him. She then lies back and
relaxes against him. He supports his weight
on his hands and draws his thighs up to
both support and encase her.. Tenderness
and torrid sex. We tend to think of them
as mutually exclusive, but they aren't.
If you take nothing else from our foray
into a non-Western way of making love,
it's that lesson.

13

TOP POSITION

tongs

You can both boost your bliss levels with an old favorite! Vatsyayana was all for women being in control.

How to do it

Nothing too fancy about this one—it's your basic woman-on-top! He lies back and relaxes, she sits on top of him, knees bent. It's called the "tongs" because instead of lifting herself up and down, she's squeezing his penis repeatedly with her vaginal muscles, moving it in and out rather like someone using a pair of tongs!

Why you'd want to

Most couples alternate between two to three positions—and this is inevitably one of them for good reason. His hands are totally free to ravish her—and it's all laid out in front of him, including a bird's-eye view of her breasts, pleasantly jiggling away. She's in complete control of penetration and can easily reach down to touch her clitoris or hold a wand vibrator for extra stimulation.

Hot hint

If her muscles aren't strong enough to do the job on their own, she can easily grind with controlled, circular movements. It feels incredibly intense at his end and she gets the clitoral pressure she needs to orgasm.

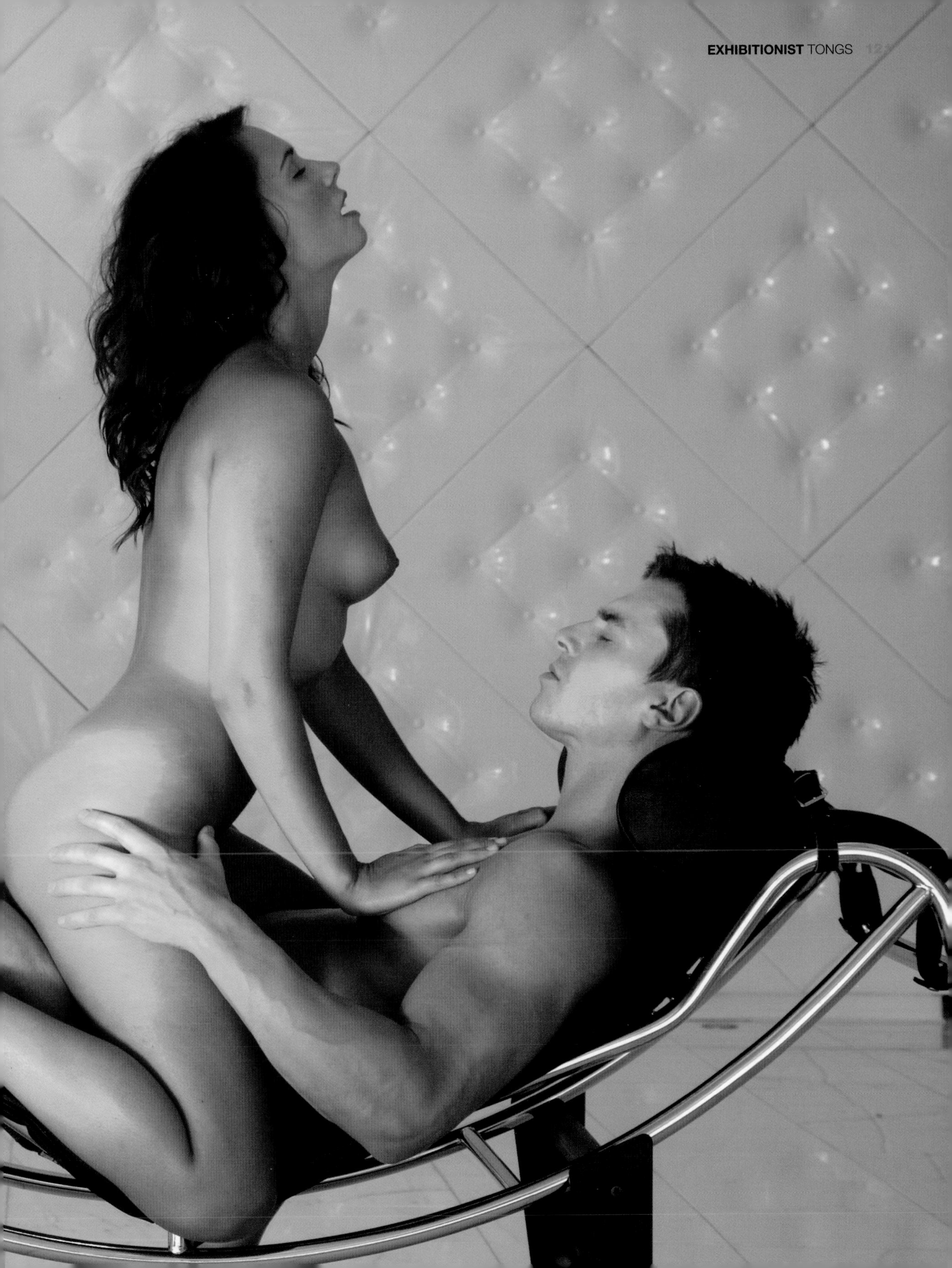

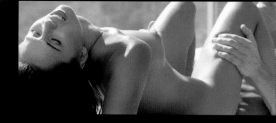

lopsided lovers

FINDING YOUR PERFECT SEXUAL PARTNER, ACCORDING TO THE ANCIENTS,
IS SIMPLY A MATTER OF MATCHING GENITAL SIZE. FIND OUT HOW YOU FARE—
AND WHAT TO DO IF YOU'RE ORGAN OPPOSITES.

She's a doe, he's a stallion (see page 113)—is finding your sexual match like star sign compatibility, where dire futures are predicted for lovers who weren't born at the right time of the year? Well, it is a bit! Vatsyayana has clear and specific instructions on who everyone's ideal sexual partner is, even if he does offer sensible suggestions if you dare to fall for the person rather than their parts.

We tend not to link **genital size with sexual compatibility**—but you don't need to be an old Indian monk to recognize that it can cause problems if the difference is extreme.

These days, we tend not to link genital size with sexual compatibility (thank God—it's hard enough finding the perfect mate without being let down at the last gate!) On the other hand, you don't need to be an old Indian monk to recognize that it can cause problems if the difference in size is extreme. Happily, whatever match you and your partner turn out to be, there's plenty you can do to even things out. All the suggestions here will make a difference—but often the biggest problem you both face isn't your genital size. It's your attitude to it. If you're completely paranoid and constantly needing reassurance, you'll be an inhibited, unadventurous lover. If your partner's the one making you feel bad, sex drains rather than boosts your self-esteem. A bigger than usual vagina doesn't suddenly render her bad in bed. A smallish penis doesn't mean he can't be a great lover. (I'm sticking by my philosophy: show me a man with a small penis, and I'll show you a man who is brilliant at oral sex!). Take differences into account, but don't focus on them.

First though, a quick reminder of who's who:
Men: from smallest to largest penis—hare, bull, stallion.
Women: from smallest to largest vagina—doe/deer, mare, elephant.

PERFECT PAIR: EQUAL UNION

Hare/doe • Bull/mare • Stallion/elephant

Since this is supposed to be the best possible match—two people with the same size parts—there's no real advice! But since sex isn't just about matching genital size, this doesn't mean you won't have a myriad of other sexual problems but hey, it's a good start!

Best positions Any and all!

SECOND BEST: HIGH UNION

Stallion/doe • Stallion/mare • Bull/doe

Basically, Vatsyayana's idea of almost-as-good intercourse, is to match men with large-ish penises with women with small-ish vaginas (in comparison to each other). While this feels great on his end (so great, in fact, premature ejaculation can become a problem), it can be painful for her under some circumstances.

Best positions Anything that doesn't allow deep penetration: man on top, side-by-side, and any position that opens her wide. Her on top is also a great choice because she's in control of penetration and speed of thrusting. Try Rising (see page 18), the Mare's position (see page 76), and Wife of Indra (see page 154).

Other tricks for him

• Only penetrate once she's fully aroused.
• Use lubricant from the start unless she's very wet, and reapply frequently if it's a long session.
• Insert your fingers first to arouse her.
• If you give her an orgasm first, through oral or manual stimulation, she'll be as lubricated and expanded as possible (not to mention happy!).
• Curb the urge to be in control of the thrusting—allow her to do it and she'll be more relaxed.

Other tricks for her

• Open your legs as wide as possible, even if your initial instinct is to close them. The average woman's vagina is 3-4 in (7–10 cm) long. When you're not aroused, the walls collapse inward. Once you're turned on, they fill with blood and the vagina swells into a balloon shape—it's smaller at the entrance. Just because it hurts at the start, doesn't mean it will continue to as he goes deeper.

• Bear down as he penetrates. It feels odd pushing out with your vaginal muscles while he's going in, but it gives you a sense of control.
• Penetrate in stages, not all in one try. Hold the base of his penis and say "OK" when he can go a little farther.
• Try him penetrating from different angles.

NOT SO GREAT: LOW UNION

Bull/elephant • Hare/elephant • Hare/mare

These are the least satisfying matches—a man with a small penis teamed with a woman with a large vagina. OK, it's not ideal, but I wouldn't be dumping each other just yet. There are loads you can do to even things up!

Best positions Think the opposite advice to that given for high union: deep penetration positions are ideal. So are positions which alter the slant of her vagina, like rear entry and her on top leaning backward. If he's on top, she should draw her knees up so they touch her chest and her feet are on his chest. Or she could put her legs on his shoulders to narrow the vaginal canal. Try the Pressed position (see page 30), and Side-by-side (see page 52)—both will shorten and narrow the yoni. Elephant (see page 40) also works.

Other tricks for him

• Don't dwell on it—choose the right position, try all the tricks, then forget about it. It's not something you can change.
• Masturbate regularly to avoid premature ejaculation, which can be common with a small penis because the nerve endings are concentrated over a smaller area.
• Give her an orgasm with your tongue or hands before you penetrate.
• Put two pillows under her bottom to alter the slant of her vagina. Thrust hard and deeply.

Other tricks for her

• Do pelvic floor exercises (see pages 72–73), start squeezing, and keep squeezing during intercourse. Contract your thigh muscles as well.
• Insert fingers or a small vibrator or dildo alongside his penis if you still don't feel "filled up."
• Keep your thighs together and get him to put his legs outside yours.

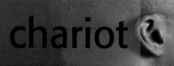

chariot

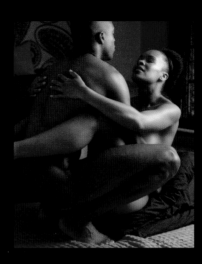

>> STEP TWO

Staying inside her, he tips her backward. She supports herself by holding onto his back, he also holds on tight. The tipping action changes the feeling for both of them, since it dramatically alters the angle of her vagina.

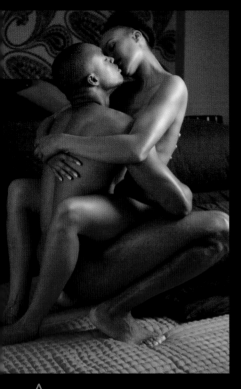

^ STEP ONE

Even though it's harder to balance on a cushy surface, it'll pay off later… believe me! He squats, she lowers herself onto his penis to sit in his lap and kiss him sexily.

>> STEP THREE

Dropping onto the soft surface, still connected, this time you both extend your legs, placing them near or on each other's shoulders, supporting your own weight on your elbows. The angle of the vaginal canal alters again, providing another novel sensation.

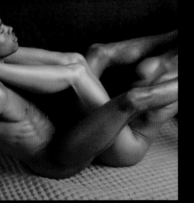

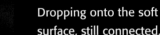

>> STEP FOUR

Sitting up to move closer, he widens his thighs as you both link arms underneath his knees. His feet are on the floor to steady you as you both move into a rocking motion. It's a balancing act, and it can quickly get to the point where maintaining the pose outweighs the pleasure

>> STEP FIVE

… And that's the moment when it makes perfect sense to shift into the infinitely more relaxing final position. Erotically knitted together, it's time to seesaw your way to orgasm. Open your eyes and watch each other climax if you want to up the intensity.

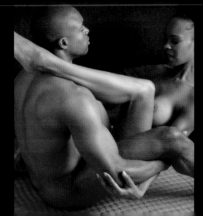

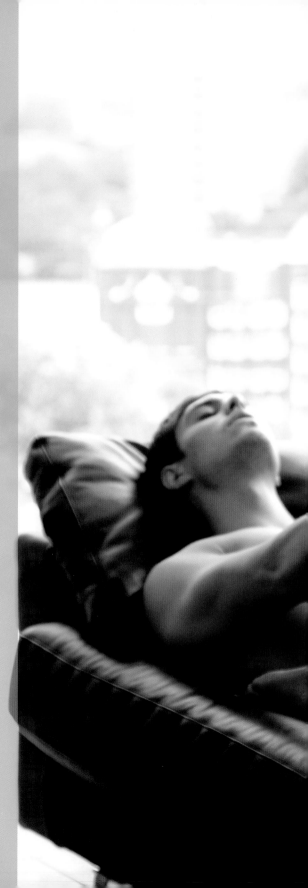

14

TOP POSITION

swing

She swings sensually from side to side for a sinfully sexy sensory treat. He gets to lie back and simply enjoy the sensation.

How to do it

He lies back, she faces his feet and lowers herself onto his penis with knees bent and calves folded back toward him. She leans onto his thighs for support—he lies back and relishes in the steamy sight of her bottom lifting up and down and swinging from side to side before him.

Why you'd want to

This one's more for him than her because there's a visual feast for him, but little in the way of clitoral stimulation. On the other hand, turning him on so much is a *huge* turn-on for her! No face-to-face contact means you can feel but not see your partner, making it fabulous for fantasies.

Hot hint

She can either sit up or—if she's feeling naughty—lean forward, resting her weight on her hands to expose both her vulva and anus. But be careful: leaning forward too enthusiastically will leave both of you feeling oddly empty. That'll be because his penis has popped out!

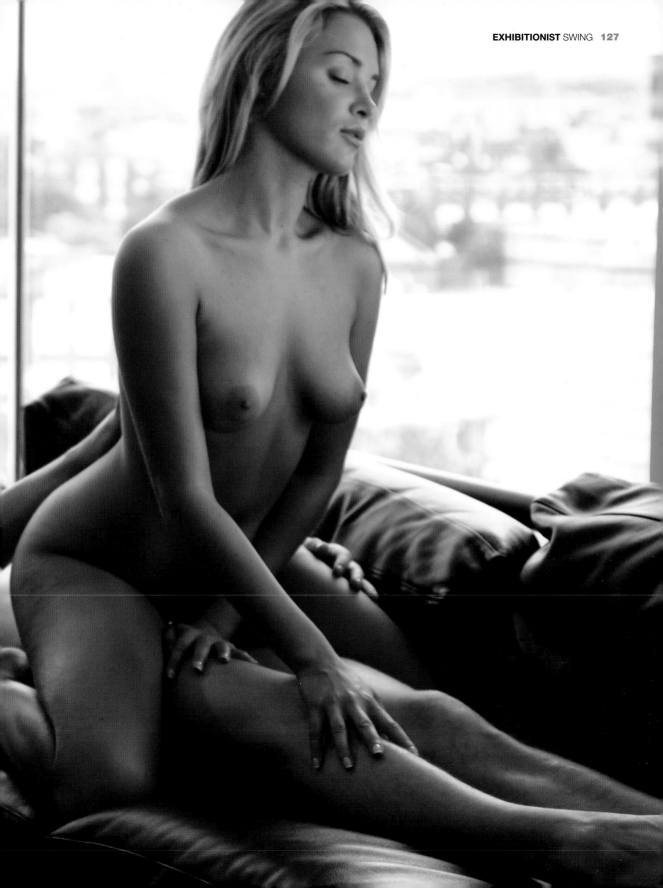

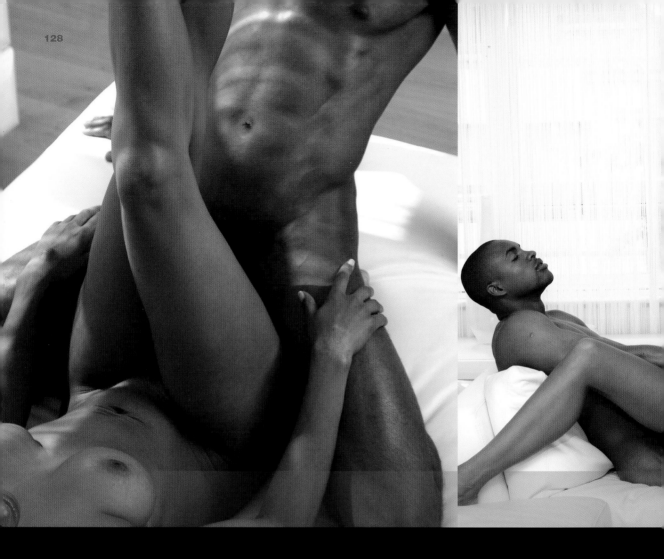

An exotic, erotic adventure

MAKE THE NEIGHBORS JEALOUS BY FORMING SEDUCTIVE SILHOUETTES THAT FEEL AS REMARKABLE AS THEY LOOK.

CROSSED LOVERS

She lies back and raises her legs straight in the air, and crosses one over the other. He penetrates and leans backward on his hands to support his weight. This is known as a "packed" position, which means her thighs are raised and placed one on top of the other. It's purported to be the most intense way a woman can grip her partner's penis with her vagina, which is why it's on your must-do List. If she contracts her vaginal muscles at the same time, his penis feels a surprisingly fierce and sexy squeeze.

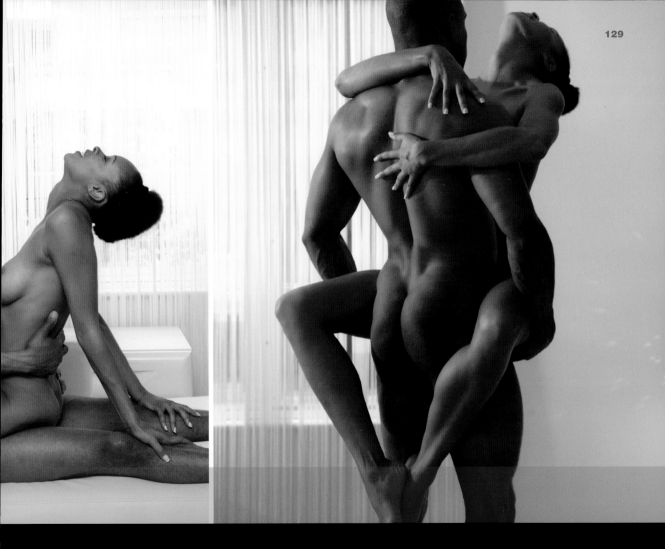

GODDESS

He sits back with lots of cushions propping
him up so he can comfortably see what's

TARZAN

She sits on the edge of a high surface
(kitchen counter?) and wraps her legs

the swivel

<< STEP ONE

Want to really impress her the first time you have sex? (Even Vatsyayana warns this one takes a lot of practice!) Pull this one off and she'll be on the phone to her girlfriends seconds after you're gone! Start in the basic missionary position but just as she's starting to think (yawn) "How predictable," you pull back, look deep into her eyes… and prepare to move.

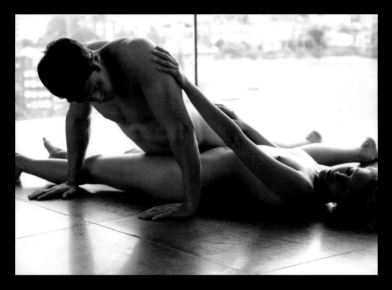

<< STEP TWO

Lift one leg, then the other so both your legs are on one side of her, being careful so your penis doesn't pop out! Keep your legs slightly apart so this doesn't happen. Work yourself around by moving your hands and feet until your body lies sideways

>> STEP THREE

Keep moving around until you're facing her toes, *very* carefully lifting one leg over her face into position. (Pray she's not squeamish because she has a prime view of a very private part!) You didn't quite get there or (worse) accidentally kicked her/fell over/fell out? Hopefully she's got a sense of humor. Better to save it until you've got it down pat.

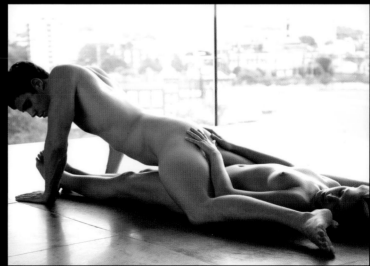

15

TOP POSITION

the vine

This one is a bit of a carnal challenge, but for fast, urgent, spontaneous sex you can't beat it.

How to do it

She leans against a wall, lifting one leg to help him penetrate and he stands between her thighs, holding her raised leg under her bottom and upper thigh. She leans into the wall for stability and to allow him to thrust away with abandon. The higher she lifts her leg on his thigh, the deeper the penetration.

Why you'd want to

For urgent, spontaneous sex, this one's a favorite. It's terribly manly with a "me Tarzan, you Jane" feel to it: he feels strong and she feels outrageously ravaged. It's also perfect for a quickie: no need to remove clothes, just hurriedly and feverishly push them aside!

Hot hint

This one's tricky if you're completely different heights. If you're having trouble getting into position, try penetrating while she's seated on the side of the bed and lifting her up from there.

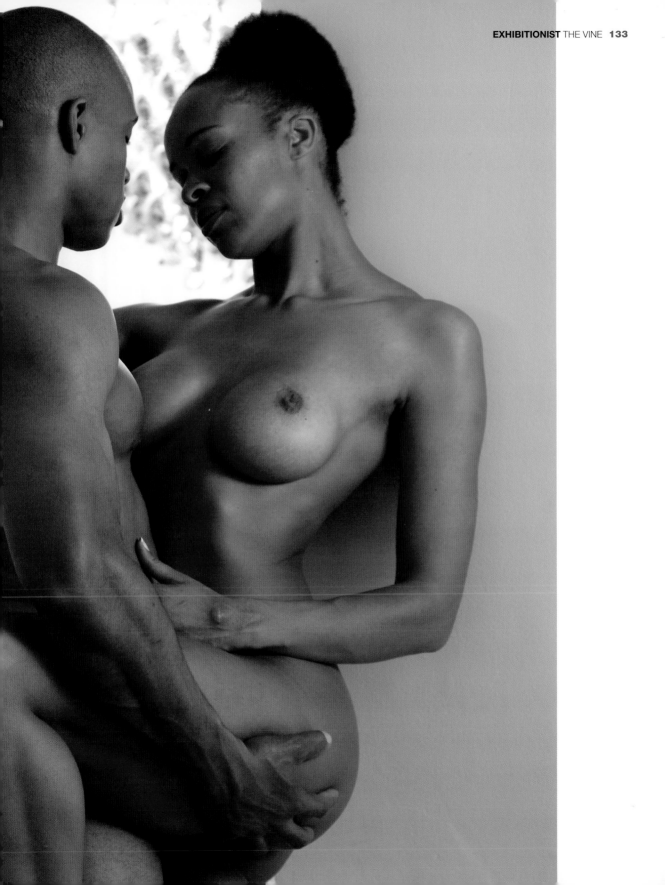

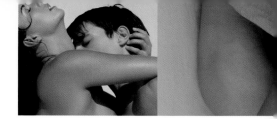

wave goodbye to ordinary orgasms

HERE'S A SNEAK PREVIEW OF THE INFAMOUS "WHOLE-BODY ORGASM" TO GET YOU TINGLING FROM TIP TO TOE. AND IF YOU'RE REALLY, REALLY GOOD, WHO SAYS YOU HAVE TO STOP AT ONE?

I'm talking purely to women here, so if you're a guy, turn to page 142 for your turn (or score big brownie points by reading on, so you can understand what she's trying to achieve). These are Tantra-inspired techniques which center on what every spiritual sex student really signs ups for: the legendary whole-body orgasm. There's a lot of hype surrounding this one: some poo-poo the whole concept, others claim it's provided the most powerful experience of their lives. The difference between a WBO and your average garden variety is you'll feel it throughout your body, not just centered in your genital area. Picture wavelike pulsations of energy surging from head to toe and you'll get some idea of what it feels like. Bring it on? I certainly will but I think you know what I'm going to say next… Yup, it takes tons of practice to master it! The first step involves learning how to circulate your "chi" (natural life energy) throughout your "microcosmic orbit"—a pathway which runs through the body. Then, using what's called an "orgasmic upward draw," you transform your sexual energy into "chi" and add it to the other "chi" to make a particularly potent brew. Yes really.

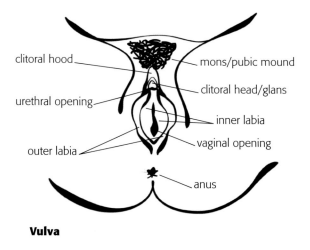

clitoral hood

mons/pubic mound

clitoral head/glans

urethral opening

inner labia

vaginal opening

outer labia

anus

Vulva

As you can imagine, this involves a hell of a lot more training than my super-simplified version. But this does give you a good idea of what you're in for—and lets you find out if you've got a natural "talent" for it. I've taken principles from the WBO and "orgasmic upward draw" and brought them right back to basics, then just to really confuse you, I've added Tantric tips on how to go on and have multiple WBOs. See how you go (or skip straight to the "cheat's version" to get the good parts).

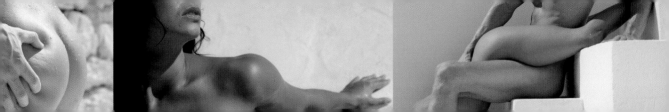

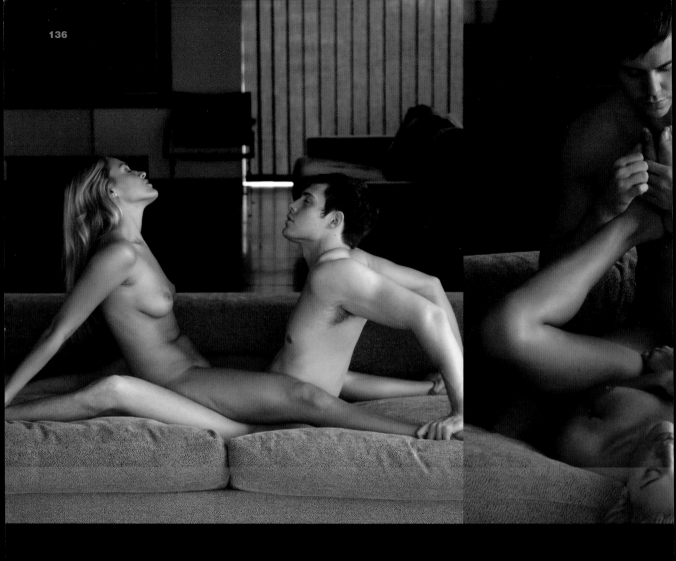

Branching out for better sex

A FOCUS ON FEET AND STRATEGIC PLACEMENT OF HER LIMBS PAYS SEXUAL DIVIDENDS FOR BOTH OF YOU.

PLAYING FOOTSIE

Clasping onto each other's feet during sex was deeply significant in ancient India. The feet are seen as highly erotic, with many drawings of men satisfying women by using their big toes to stimulate the clitoris. This position is designed to allow both of you to hold and massage each other's feet—and to provide a tranquil pose for you to lie still and/or circulate the sexual energy that's passing between you. If instead you find yourself bringing up what color to paint the walls, it's time to move on.

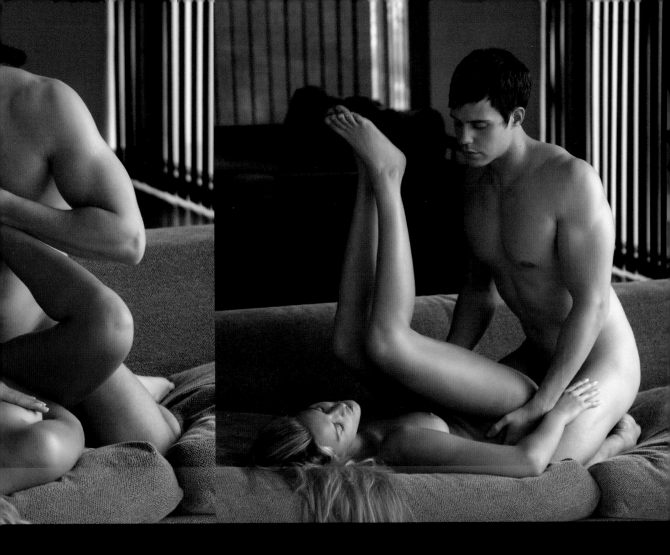

PICTURE FRAME

She lies back and he kneels in front of her. He takes hold of her feet and brings the soles together, pushing her legs back toward her chest. Her legs then form a triangular shape, forming a "frame" around both your genital areas. Sweet and spiritually significant—but there are some purely practical reasons for giving this one a try. For a start, it gives her easy access to her clitoris, upping the odds of her climaxing in this position. Secondly, she can play with her own breasts, making *his* day!

THE ALL-ROUNDER

She stays lying down and drops her legs back toward her head, exposing her vagina and pushing her labia invitingly toward him. If you're aiming for her to have multiple orgasms in one session, this is a good position to be in because it's easy for him to move from penetration to giving her oral sex and on to anal play and manual stimulation with his fingers. Alternating between different types of stimulation gives her the best chance of climaxing more than once.

16

TOP POSITION

crab

This is satisfyingly show-off, but also relatively simple. Send each other into erotic overdrive—in comfort!

How to do it

She lies back and pulls her knees up to her chin. He kneels in front and penetrates, holding onto the front of her calves to hold them together and for balance. She can hold onto his upper thighs to help provide leverage.

Why you'd want to

This position gives super*super*deep penetration so make sure it's not a "sensitive cervix" day (don't laugh, it really can be influenced by what time of the month it is!). It's a raw, primitive position which tends to lead to quick orgasms, hopefully for both of you! Her legs are together which means a tighter, shallower vaginal canal; he's thrusting straight down instead of at an angle which directly hits her front vaginal wall.

Hot hint

It's hard work on your legs and you both may feel the need to stretch them out at some point. Switch to this one when you're both on the edge of orgasm or use it as an erotic appetizer.

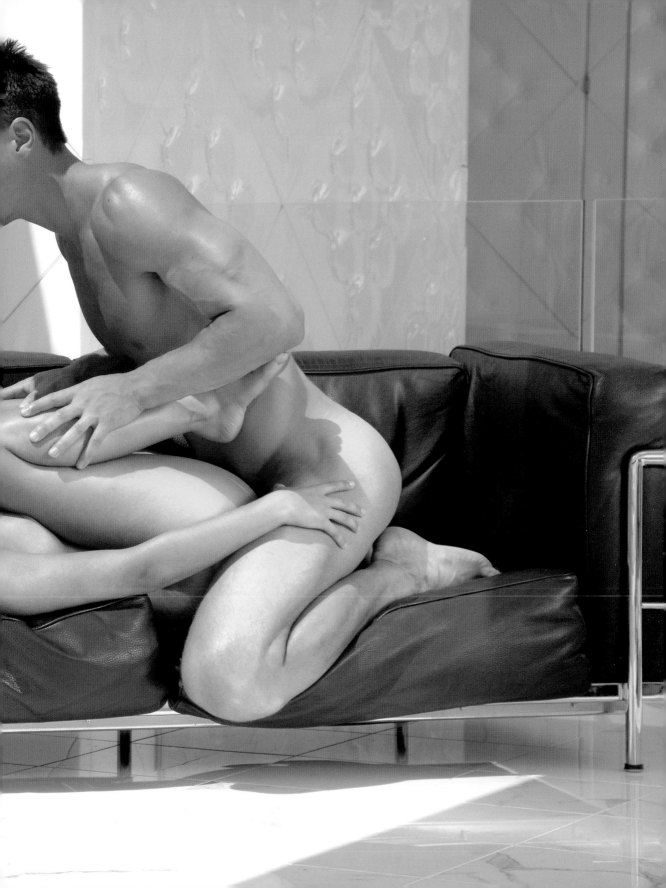

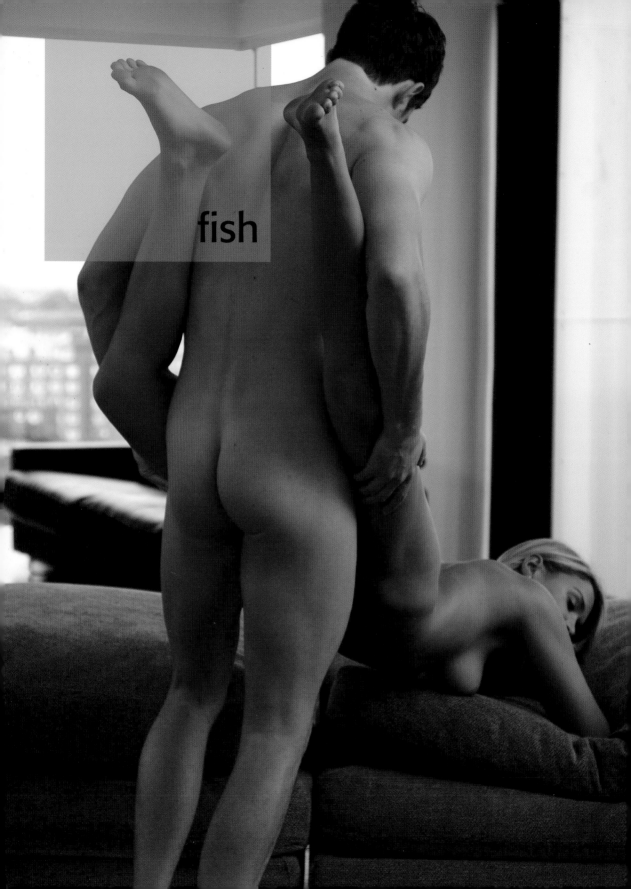

fish

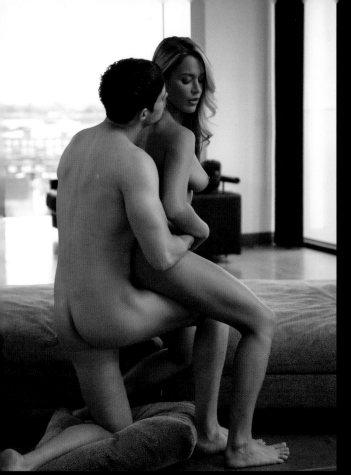

<< STEP ONE

Vatsyayana often looked to animals to get inspiration for positions and techniques. This, he claims, will make her feel like she's swimming. (Did people do drugs back then?) He kneels, rather sensibly, on a cushion with one leg raised. She takes a seat, lowering herself onto his penis. He enjoys a pit stop to play with her clitoris, fondle her breasts, kiss her neck, and generally ravish her!

STEP TWO

She leans forward, resting her forearms on a piece of furniture. He holds her by the waist and starts thrusting gently. If you're planning on trying the Sets of Nine (see page 153),
V now's the time!
V

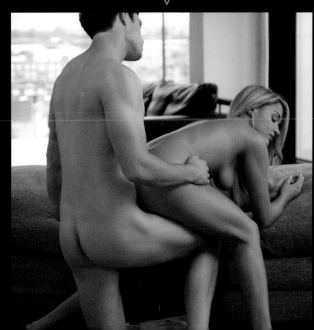

<< STEP THREE

He stands up, not without some difficulty (if he didn't start with strong legs, he'll sure as hell sport bulging thigh muscles when we're finished!), taking a firm hold of her upper thighs. She's now completely supporting her weight on her elbows and forearms, and braces herself as he moves into deep, passionate thrusting. Feel like a fish? Didn't think so.

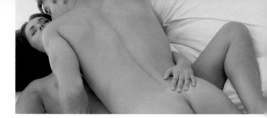

cosmic coming

WANT AN ORGASM THAT EXPLODES IN YOUR HEAD... BUT LEAVES YOU NICE AND HARD AND READY FOR ROUND TWO? LIKE DEEPER, EXPLOSIVE CONTRACTIONS AND BEING A MASTER OF EJACULATION? SHE'S HAD HERS, NOW IT'S YOUR TURN...

According to Taoists, there are four stages of erection: firmness, swelling, hardness, and heat. The last part—when the testicles draw close to your body to make sure semen is the right temperature for fertilization—is the part we're trying to avoid. (Unless of course your partner is desperately trying to get pregnant, in which case, delaying ejaculation is the last thing you need!) Here's the second part you have to come to grips with: not only are orgasm and ejaculation two different processes (the first is pleasure registered in your brain, the second is the physical release of semen), there are two stages of ejaculation. During the *contractile* stage, the prostate gland contracts and empties semen into the urethra. It's only during the *expulsion* stage that semen is ejected down the urethra and out of the pelvis. The general idea is to let the first part happen, but not the second. You might think it's all out of your control, but Taoists believe ejaculation is voluntary. All you need to do is squeeze your PC muscle and you'll draw the blood and energy your body needs to ejaculate, away from the organs. (And no, it's not bad for you!)

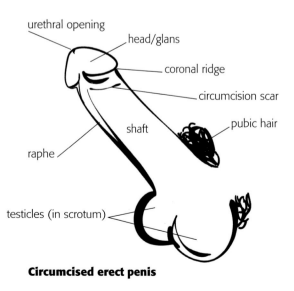

urethral opening

head/glans

coronal ridge

circumcision scar

pubic hair

shaft

raphe

testicles (in scrotum)

Circumcised erect penis

But before you start, a word on the stopping ejaculation part: you've got about as much chance of controlling ejaculation the first few times you try this as mastering Latin on your lunch hour. Like, it ain't going to happen. Even Mantak Chia, the master of multiple orgasms himself, admits it's like "trying to stop a team of horses who are speeding toward a cliff." So why even try? Well, once you get it right you'll not only feel an incredibly invigorating rush of energy, you can boast to the guys about your supreme control—and impress the hell out of her!

CLIMAX WITHOUT CONCLUSION

There are lots of techniques that claim to delay ejaculation, this one's called "The Big Draw." The basic idea is for you to stop thrusting when you feel close to orgasm (no surprise there!). The "Big Draw" partly refers to you moving energy up through your body and using it to keep those pelvic floor muscles strong so you can control ejaculation (which is a *little* out there but, you've got to admit, sounds logical!).

If you decide the "proper" version isn't for you, at least read it. There are lots of cool tricks to be gleaned and the "cheat's version" makes more sense if you read all of it. Try this one on your own first.

The basics
• Masturbate till you've got a seriously hard erection, but aren't about to orgasm. Stop, wait for a minute, then contract your anus and pelvic floor muscle (see page 72) firmly and clamp your toes to the floor.
• Inhale and draw the sexual energy you've created away from your perineum (the bit between your anus and testicles) and anus, toward your spine. Do this by squeezing your bottom cheeks together tightly.
• At the same time, move into a pumping motion, so you're squeezing and relaxing your PC muscle.
• Tuck your chin in to allow the energy to move into your skull and roll your eyes up to pull it to the crown of your head. (Handy tip: a locked door between you and the rest of the house is a brilliant idea.)
• You're successful if you look down and your erection has… well, sort of gone. Granted, this isn't usually a time for celebration, but in the "Big Draw" it is. The person with the limpest penis gets the gold star.
• Repeat the process (from the part where you contract your muscles) a total of nine times.

Now, here's where we get a bit hippy-trippy, so hang on to your happy pants…
• Keep masturbating until you feel yourself in the *contractile* stage, contractions in your prostate lasting about 3–5 seconds (it takes a lot of practice to

recognize this). Hold perfectly still until you regain control of your arousal (to stop it from tipping over into *expulsion*), then immediately try spiraling…
• During spiraling you use your mind, eyes, and all your senses to spiral the sexual energy you created into your brain—up to 36 times. That's right, you're tossing it first in one direction, then the other. Get this right and you've just had the equivalent of a "mental orgasm" (that's one you feel in the brain rather than one that's a bit crazy and silly).
• When your brain feels "full," touch your tongue to the roof of your mouth and allow the energy to flow down your body to the navel where it can be safely stored.
• Now look down and what a surprise… your penis may still be erect! If you don't ejaculate, you don't lose your erection. So you're ready for round two… There! It's that easy! Not. Interested in more? Get a copy of Mantak Chia's *The Multi-Orgasmic Man*.

The cheat's version
• Masturbate until you're highly aroused, then stop, hold still, and contract your PC muscle *hard*. The stronger your love muscle, the more control you'll have over it. Squeeze away while you're watching TV/football/asking for a raise/flirting with that girl.
• Concentrate on keeping your heart rate as low as possible. Your body associates ejaculation with a thudding, "Jeez-this-is-nice!" type heartbeat. Slowing it down tricks your body and brain. Do this by breathing slowly and calmly.
• Start masturbating after a few moments and repeat the whole process a couple of times. Imagine you're drawing the sexual energy up your spine, and away from your genitals.
• As you feel yourself hit 8–9 on a scale of 1–10 for orgasm (10 being lift off), stop, contract your PC again—visualize the energy shooting to your brain.
• If you feel an orgasm explode in your head but look down to see you've still got an erection, log on to my website and ask me out. (Only kidding—really!)

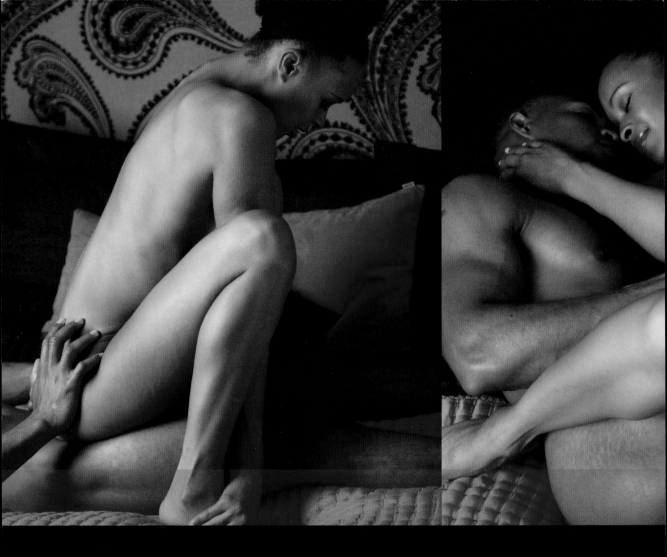

Twist and tilt for a fresh feel

SURPRISINGLY SUBTLE CHANGES IN DIFFERENT BODY PARTS CAN MAKE A BIG DIFFERENCE TO HOW A POSITION LOOKS AND FEELS.

THE STRETCH

He lies on his back, she turns her back on him and lowers herself onto his penis in a sitting position. Grasping her feet, she then pulls herself upward so her torso is as straight as possible. Back in *Kama Sutra* time, an ancient Indian man would then have admired her elegance, flexibility, and superior posture. Today, he's more likely to be checking out how good her bottom looks going up and down on his penis. She's supposed to do all the thrusting, but he can help by lifting her at the hips.

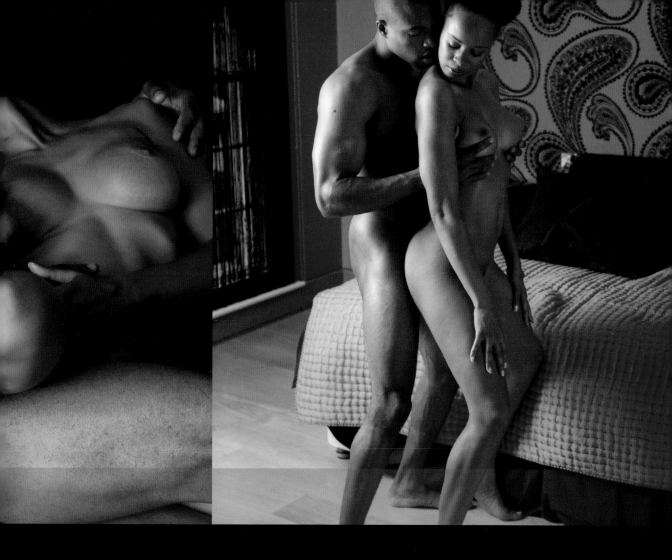

THE TWIST

This position looks awkward because she's twisted but it's actually surprisingly relaxing. Start by both lying on your sides and penetrate as you usually would in a side-by-side position. At this point you're both facing in the same direction. She then lifts her top leg, winding it backward over his waist and thigh. You can hold hands and if she puts her other hand up to hold his face, this can be super-romantic as well as sexy. Go with the mood. Don't be scared to turn what's supposed to be a lusty position into a loving one, or vice versa.

THE TILT

Don't even attempt this one unless you're at least comparable in height. (Or wear high heels to even it up!) She also needs flexible hips because she has to tilt her bottom up and backward. The wider she spreads her legs, the easier it becomes, but although placing her hands on her thighs gives some stability, if he's thrusting vigorously, it's fairly easy to topple over! So why bother? He can touch her breasts, clitoris, perineum—it's virtually all reachable—making all the effort on her part (almost) worth it.

17

TOP POSITION

the nail

More playful than passionate, this is perfect for a lighthearted romp. Try taking sex seriously with someone's foot on your head!

How to do it

Officially called "fixing a nail," the name is inspired by her placing her heel on his forehead—the idea being, her calf and foot look like a hammer, his head resembles the head of a nail. Hmmm. Sounds a bit dangerous to me, but I'm liking the leg in the air bit! It's cute and quirky and simple to do: she lies flat, he kneels astride her and penetrates. She then stretches one leg out and lifts the other, putting her foot into position.

Why you'd want to

In this position the thrusting has to be slow and controlled, which can be unbearably sexy. To up the erotic tension, he can put his hand on her breastbone and pretend to hold her down. Be warned though: while some women find this a deliciously "dangerous" turn-on, others may feel uncomfortable or threatened.

Hot hint

As he thrusts, her leg moves. If the thought of her kicking you in the face doesn't really appeal, get her to put her leg to the side. Even better, suck her toes.

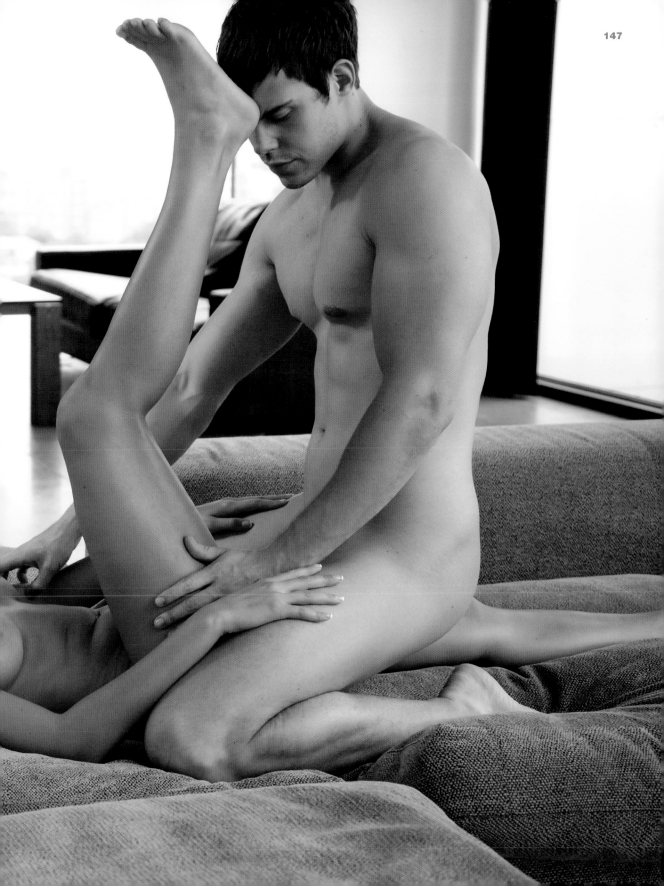

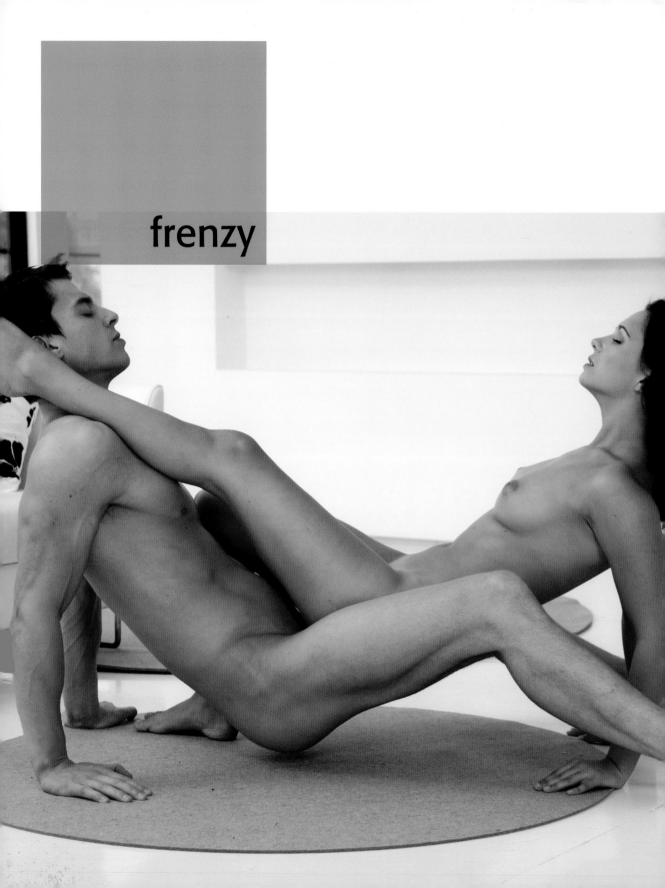

frenzy

<< STEP ONE

You're either flexing those well-toned and honed muscles of yours or rolling around laughing after taking a look at this one. You need to be strong, supple, and yoga fit to last longer than a few minutes. But hey, big points for trying! It starts off simply enough: he sits with straight legs and penetrates as she climbs on top.

STEP TWO

As he holds onto her waist, supporting her, she leans back, taking her weight on her hands. She then puts (and leaves) one foot on the floor and rests the other leg on his shoulder.

V
V

<< STEP THREE

In the final move, he lets her go so she's totally supporting her own weight and moves his hands into a mirror position. Keeping both feet on the ground, he pushes up on his arms and thrusts his hips upward to create movement. It's a novel sensation and you both feel terribly smug for a bit, having managed it. Then your arms hurt. Then you notice your belly jiggling. Then you collapse, quickly moving into an old favorite to finish the job.

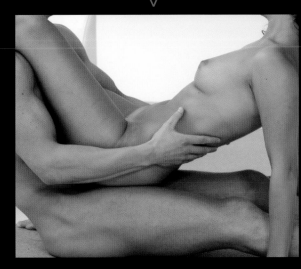

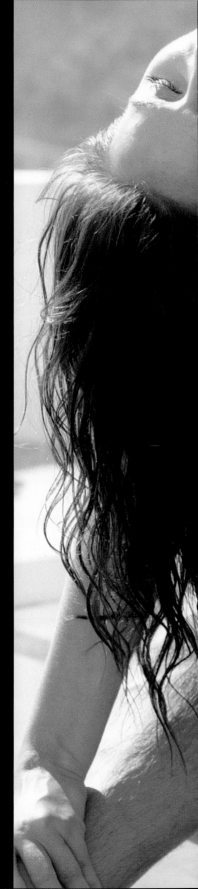

erotic

exotic

xhilarating

xhibitionist

expert

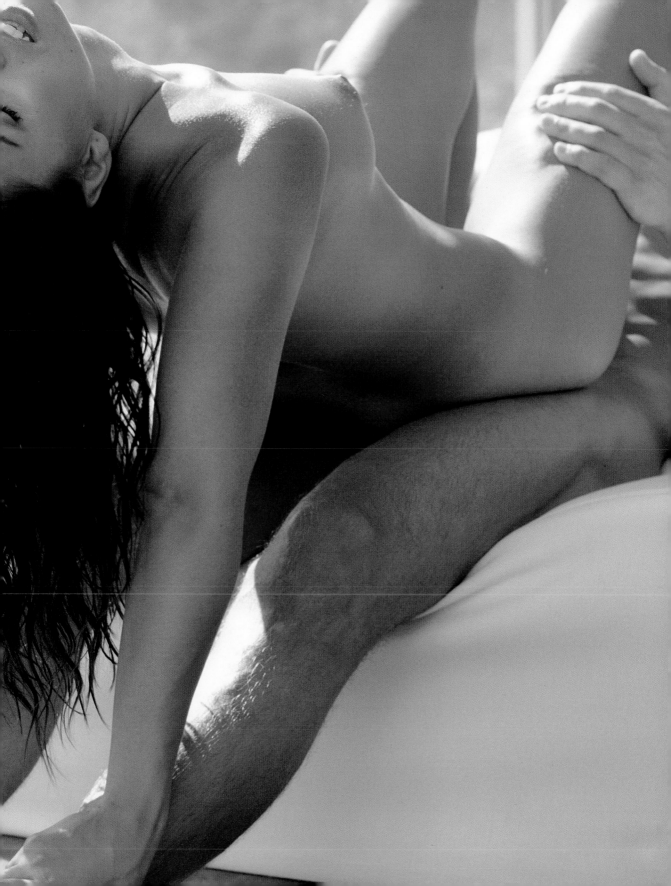

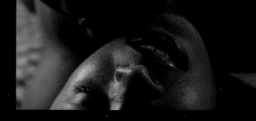

take the plunge

WHY VATSYAYANA WAS A CLOSET FEMINIST AND WHY WOMEN SHOULD JUMP ON TOP FOR BETTER ORGASMS. THE PAIR OF TONGS, THE SWING, AND THE BEE ARE ALL TECHNIQUES GUARANTEED TO GET YOU BOTH BUZZING!

Forget what the history books tell you, in the *Kama Sutra* sexual equality existed 2,000 years ago. Yes, there are some sections in there that smack of sexism, but there's one hell of a lot in it that empowers women. Vatsyayana portrays females as sensual, sexual beings who are able to—and should—initiate and take control during sex.

A prime purpose of the *Kama Sutra* is to teach men to be sensitive, skillful lovers who understand the sexual needs of women. Vatsyayana realized the female sexual system was different than a man's—and he recognized that women are more instinctive about sex than men, needing less formal instruction because of our strongly developed sense of intuition. Most importantly, the *Kama Sutra* teaches women not to be ashamed of sex or desire. And let's face it, that's a pretty big deal since shame about sex is *still* being used to control women even now! Yes, it was a book written about sex for men so it sounds sexist. In reality, it's anything but.

The ultimate aim is to keep it inside for 100 heartbeats. Since both your hearts will be thudding away like crazy, this isn't as long as it sounds.

For instance, her hopping on top to take control—both of penetration (and her orgasm) is perfectly OK. In fact, if you notice he's a tad tuckered out, Vatsyayana positively encourages it! You're supposed to ask permission first, of course (sorry did someone say something?), but then feel free to turn him onto his back and go for it sister! Other permitted reasons to take the "male role," besides fatigue, include curiosity or a simple hankering to do something different. Thought you'd get to lie back while he did all the work? Hah! You've obviously never read any of my books before.

THRUSTING FOR HER

The next time you're on top (yes, it does mean effort, but trust me, it pays off!) try fast or slow rocking, moving your hips in slow circles, and raising or lowering on to him at different speeds. If you mix up your thrusting style, the average bout of intercourse is going to be one hell of a lot more interesting. It not only makes you look sexually savvy and erotically experienced, it ups your chance of having an orgasm through penetration only, and feels damn good for him, too. Try all of the following:

The (pair of) tongs Clench your PC muscles (having toned them to perfection doing the exercises on page 73) and hold his penis inside you as tight as you possibly can. Grip, squeeze, and internally stroke it by "milking" (think the rhythmic ritual of milking a cow—squeeze and release, squeeze and release). The ultimate aim is to keep it inside for 100 heartbeats. Since both your hearts will be thudding away like crazy, this isn't as long as it sounds.

The top You turn around on the man's body like a wheel so that your back is toward him. Yes, this isn't one to be tackled half-heartedly. Think lots of practice, giggles, and training and you're about one-fifth there.

The bee Crouch in a sitting position over him and revolve your vagina around his penis while he arches his back to make it easier. "Easier" said with tongue-in-cheek: this is an advanced technique (but it's not so far out there that you shouldn't attempt it!)

The swing Sway in wide circles over him, using your whole body to make a figure of eight. Again, ambitious but doable—give it a go!

Melting together When you feel tired of being the boy, lie down on top of him and rest without breaking coital contact. (Thought you'd like this one—I can hear you sighing!) That's the whole point of spiritual sex—there's no reason to rush. Yes, the *Kama Sutra* was written when school car pools and morning meetings didn't exist, but it won't kill you to pause for a few minutes. To get things going again, move gently to restimulate his penis and the two of you.

NINE THRUSTS TO NIRVANA

The sets of nine is a set of thrusting movements based around nine sets. However simplistic this technique sounds, it does revitalize sex-weary, worn-out genitals by thoroughly massaging the vagina and nudging the penis into "wake up and pay attention" mode. As a Taoist technique, its true purpose is the flow of energy between you. Less lofty types will like it simply because it's fun and something new to try. It was originally intended to have him on top. I'm reversing that, so the female is in charge, for several reasons. First up, men take the lead role in thrusting around 90 percent of the time. If we truly want sexual equality (and we do!) women need to become more active during sex. Secondly, women who jump on top have more orgasms. Why? You can angle his penis to hit the front vaginal wall and/or squat so your clitoris rubs against the base of his penis. Get it right and you could experience two orgasms for the price of one!

Here's the basic formula. Try to resist the urge to count out loud (or count in sexy, gutteral tones if you do!):
• Nine shallow, one deep.
• Eight shallow, two deep.
• Seven shallow, three deep.
• Six shallow, four deep.
• Five shallow, five deep.
• Four shallow, six deep.
• Three shallow, seven deep.
• Two shallow, eight deep.
• One shallow, nine deep.

Try to go through as many sets as possible without him ejaculating. In reality, you'll both probably get bored/and or confused after the third round of four shallow, six deep (or was it six shallow, four deep, yikes!). But don't worry—it's more about understanding the principle than following it to a tee.

If you grasp nothing else but that you should mix thrusting up and contrast deep with shallow strokes, rather than sticking to the usual in-out maneuver, you're a step ahead of where you were.

18

TOP POSITION

wife of indra

Spiritualists say sex is food both for the body and the soul. So try this one for a fabulously frisky feast!

How to do it

She lies back pulling her knees up to her chin, and he kneels in front and penetrates. She then rests her feet on his chest, using it to give her enough leverage to lift her bottom into the air.

Why you'd want to

This one's all about her squeezing those (by now beautifully toned) pelvic floor muscles. I know you're sick of hearing it, but it's the basis of many of the positions and techniques of spiritual sex. And it has a *huge* effect on how good intercourse feels for both of you. So stop complaining and start squeezing! Certain positions, like this one, make it easier for her to tense and contract. Indra, by the way, was a Hindu god and this position is named after his (very seductive) wife!

Hot hint

You need a certain height difference for this to work well, so use cushions to even things up if needed. Oh—and take a tip from the couple pictured and save your knees from carpet burn by doing it on a soft surface.

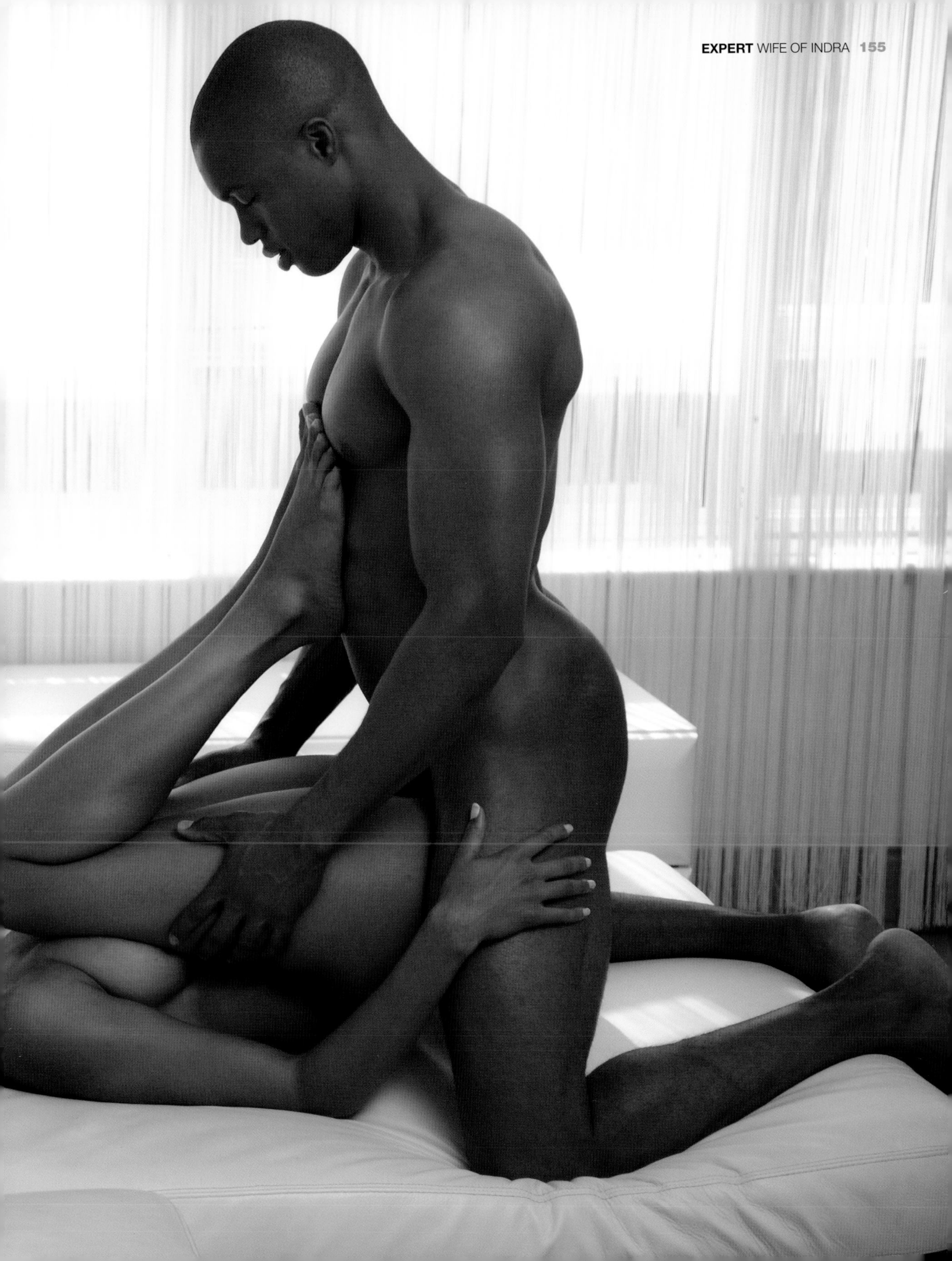

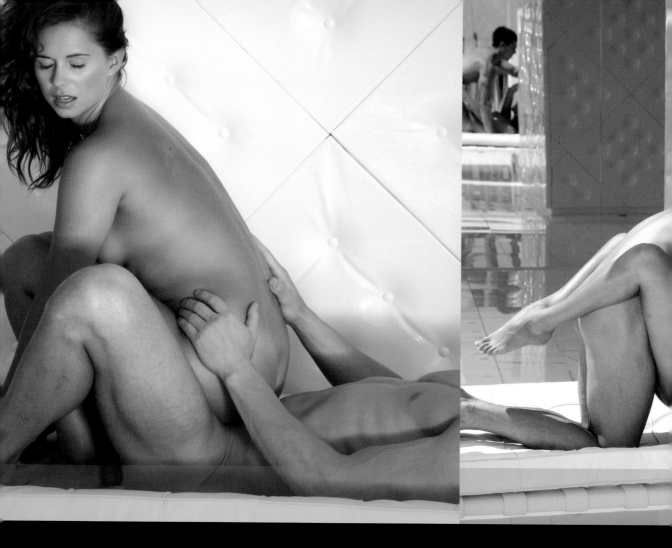

Flashy positions for frisky lovers

HANG ONTO YOUR HEADBOARD BECAUSE WE'RE NOW MOVING INTO BOAST-ABOUT POSITIONS YOU *WON'T* BE TRYING AFTER A BEER AT THE BAR.

FANTASY FODDER

Want to make intercourse last longer? This position is a good option because thrusting is limited on his part. The less intense the friction, the less likely he is to ejaculate early. He lies down and she sits facing away from him. There's no eye contact and little body contact, which makes it seem impersonal for some. But if you're in the mood for living out a lurid fantasy that *doesn't* revolve around your partner, this becomes a plus! (It's normal to fantasize about people other than your partner, by the way!)

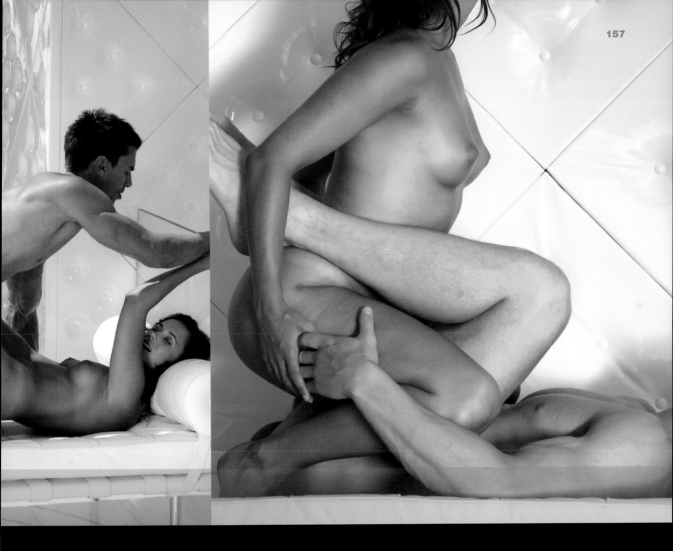

GET A GRIP

One question before we start: do you dance well together? If the answer is no, it's probably best if you skip this because it's all about couple coordination. She lies back, legs parted and grips the headboard with one hand. He kneels between her legs and penetrates, she grips her legs around his hips and allows herself to be pulled upward as he leans forward to also hold onto the back of the bed. You then move into a seesaw motion, using your hands to pull and push against the headboard.

THE HORSE RIDE

This position is inspired by horse riding: he lies on his back and draws his knees up, parting his thighs. She wiggles between them, using her hand to help insert his penis, then leans forward, using her knees to move up and down on his penis, "riding" him like he's a horse. (Hopefully he's just as well hung). Putting firm cushions under his shoulders can make this easier. If her legs start to get tired (which is absolutely in the cards), he can sit up while she sits back so you're sitting face to face.

19

TOP POSITION

monkey

The ultimate quickie position, this is a pleasure pick-me-up which feels as dynamic as it looks.

How to do it

Standing positions feature strongly in the *Kama Sutra*, with some resembling erotic sculptures rather than intercourse positions! He leans against a wall and lifts her up by taking a firm grip of her bottom. She winds her arms around his neck, grips his thighs with hers, and puts her feet against the wall to give leverage and help him thrust. Thrusting becomes more of an up-and-down bobbing than an in-and-out motion.

Why you'd want to

Perfect for fast, passionate, impromptu sex, it's another one of those manly, caveman type positions. Yes, it's a challenge but as long as you don't expect it to last longer than a few minutes, it's totally doable!

Hot hint

The closer you are in height, the easier this position will be. Though, if you can find stairs near a wall, you might be able to even up the height difference that way. If he's shorter, he can stand on something (very) stable.

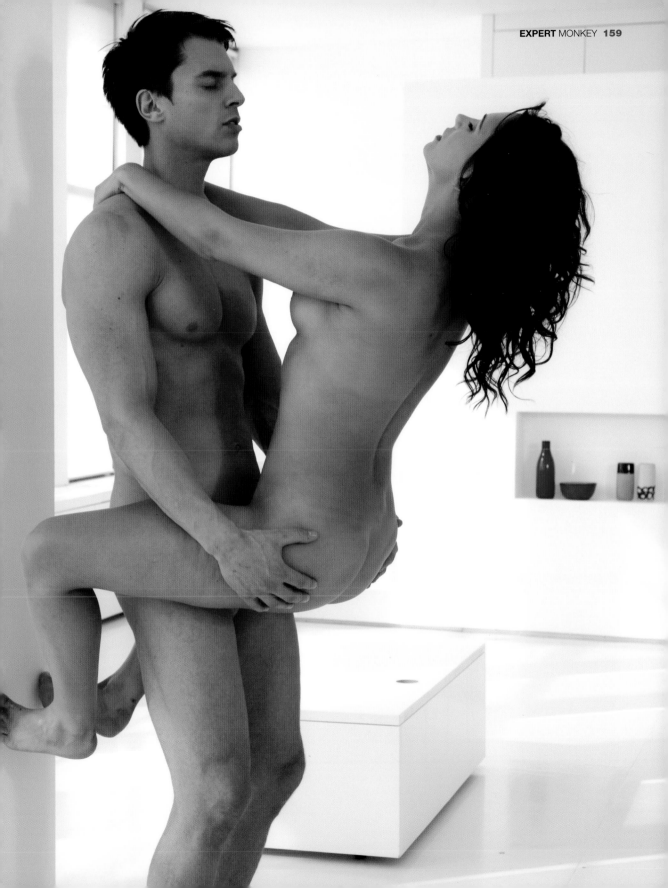

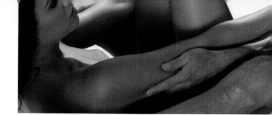

get your teeth into it

NOT SO SPIRITUAL SEX—WHY THE *KAMA SUTRA* ENCOURAGES YOU TO HURT THE ONE YOU LOVE. EVERYTHING FROM A HARMLESS "HALF MOON" TO "BITING OF THE BOAR"—ONE HELL OF A BITE! ALL YOU NEED TO KNOW TO CAUSE PLEASURABLE PAIN.

How times have changed. In *Kama Sutra* time, leaving scratches, bites, or other marks of passion in a place where everyone could see them, was very much the done thing. A stamp of sexual ownership telling the world a woman is spoken for (how boring is the modern version—wedding rings—in contrast!). "Even when a stranger sees at a distance a young woman with the marks of nails on her breast, he is filled with love and respect for her," writes Vatsyayana. Hmm. These days, he'd be more likely to think "weirdo!" Turning up at work with a whopping great love-bite on your neck isn't recommended as a great career move either. But in Vatsyayana's time, marking was not only a way of ensuring nobody stole what was yours (the whole "If you love someone set them free" thing wasn't huge back then), it was designed to give your lover something to remember you by while you're gone, evoking not just hot flashes of lust, but love.

Biting, particularly for women, was encouraged as a way to show their partner they really were enjoying themselves, rather than faking it. Though, as Vatsyayana points out—it was usually women "of a passionate nature" who did it and it was more likely to happen on certain occasions: the first time a couple have sex, before they're about to be parted, when they're reunited, during "make up" sex—and (wait for it) if a woman is drunk. (That'd be every Friday night then!)

Whichever way you look at it, scratching and biting is animalistic—which means lusty types will love it and the more timid will find it horribly intimidating. I'd say it's safe to assume most people *won't* really want to advertise what they did the night before by being marked in a place on view. But if you're talking doing it in a private place where only they can see it, well, that can be absurdly erotic. To the public, you present as Mr. or Mrs. Professional—knowing there's a huge bite on your breast as evidence of private passion is a huge aphrodisiac.

LEAVING YOUR MARK

Vatsyayana says the armpit, throat, breasts, lips, thighs, and genitals are the spots most suited to marking or scratching. If you're having *super*-hot sex, however, he graciously grants permission to do it wherever the hell you like. A few (rather obvious) rules if you want to try this out on your partner: make sure they're happy to be marked, agree on where is off limits, and only do it when they're *über* turned on. A bite out of the blue will get you slapped rather than kissed. As the *Kama Sutra* warns, "If you're having an affair, it's better to leave no trace of love marks, except in most hidden of places" (no-brainer). And make sure you don't get too carried away: don't break the skin or draw blood!

MARKS

• **Sounding** Simply dragging your nails across your lover's skin to make the hairs stand up. This should be done on the breasts and thighs.

• **Half moon** Push your nails into their skin making a crescent-shaped mark. Use this technique on their neck, breast, or chest.

• **A line** Draw your nails down the back.

• **Tiger claw** A scratch resembling a tiger claw which curves over the surface of her breast.

• **Peacock's foot** You'll need to practice this one (though it has to be said you need to get out a bit more if you really intend on doing just that!). The idea is to draw a curved line on the breast using all five fingers so it looks like a peacock's foot. I, too, am trying to conjure up an image of a peacock's foot.

• **Rabbit jump** When five marks are left close together on the breast, usually bunched up around the nipple. Good luck.

BITES

There are eight different kinds of bites used on different parts of the body. As the *Kama Sutra* says, "If variety is sought in all the arts and amusements, how much more should it be sought after in the art of love?" Exactly.

• **The hidden bite** Your classic love bite in a hidden place on the neck, breast, or chest.

• **The swollen bite** The skin is pressed down on both sides, so there's a lump.

• **The point** A nip taken with just two teeth.

• **The line of points** Small bits of skin bitten with all the teeth.

• **Coral and jewel** Biting with your teeth and using pressure from your lips on their cheek or bottom cheek. (I'd be going for the second option if I was you.) Lips are perceived as coral and the teeth as jewels.

• **The line of jewels** Biting using all your teeth.

• **The broken cloud** Done on the breast, this involves creating unevenly raised marks in a circle by sucking the skin into the space between your teeth

• **Biting of the boar** Not surprisingly, since it basically involves literally taking a piece out of your partner, this is only done by and to people of great passion. Horny little suckers in other words. Imagine a mark caused by a row of teeth, usually left on the shoulder or breast.

BLOWS

The idea of using force or violence to enhance sex isn't new to us. Spanking, tie-up games, acting out pretend "rape" scenarios, mock fighting—all are reasonably commonplace. And just as spanking a lover as sex play is eons away from hitting them in anger, the ritualized blows Vatsyayana suggests are harmless and designed to simply increase the flow of adrenalin, which turns us on and heightens excitement. You do them either before or during intercourse and there are four kinds: using the back of the hand, using slightly bent fingers, the fist, and the palm of the hand. Both men and women are encouraged to use them on the shoulders, head, the space between the breasts, back, midriff, and on the sides. Personally, the only one I'd be suggesting is the palm of the hand to the buttocks—a playful spank—but, as always, it's each to his own.

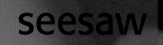

seesaw

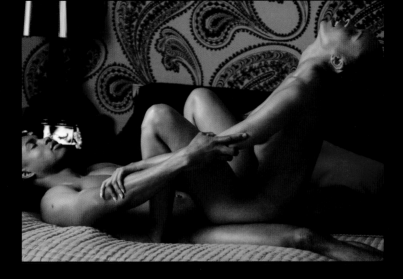

STEP ONE

He lies flat, thighs slightly parted. She plonks herself on top (or delicately climbs astride, depending on her personality), sitting erect as you grasp each other's arms. She balances by keeping her feet pressed to his sides, then slowly lets her head fall back. Stay there for a few minutes so she can get used to the feeling of blood rushing to her head during intercourse.

>> STEP TWO

She moves into position (with silent thanks for sticking to that punishing sit-up routine!) Pulling her tummy muscles tight—and keeping them clenched— helps immeasurably to pull her up and down. As well as leaning backward, she moves her feet higher on his body, wedging them against him for support. Both hold each other's wrists firmly.

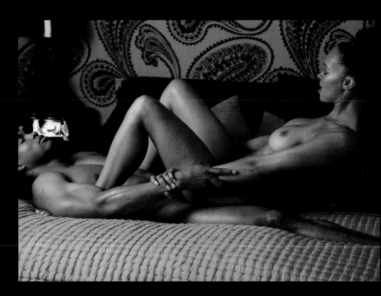

<< STEP THREE

In the final stage, she leans totally back and you both move into a rocking motion. He's pulling her back and forth using his arms; she's using her tummy muscles and her arms. You work together rather than one leading, trying to find a natural balance point. Devotees claim "upside-down" orgasms feel fantastic because the rush of blood to the head makes everything more intense. Others just end up with one hell of a headache.

20

TOP POSITION

yawning

Designed to do everything *but* make you yawn, in this position she surrenders entirely to him.

How to do it

She lies back and spreads her legs as far apart as possible. He kneels in front and penetrates, holding her ankles to hold her legs wide (and make it even sexier!)

Why you'd want to

The payoff isn't so much penetration, but her surrendering completely to him. The wider she opens herself, the more she offers her sexual soul to her lover. It's a visual vulval feast for him and it also lends itself to intense eye gazing. He can stop thrusting occasionally to lean forward and kiss her deeply; she can vary the sensation by moving the position of each leg at a time.

Hot hint

Think of this one as more of a treat for the imagination than the bod. There's no clitoral stimulation but it's such an erotic pose, you'll be happy to relinquish it. She needs to be fairly supple in the groin and hips.

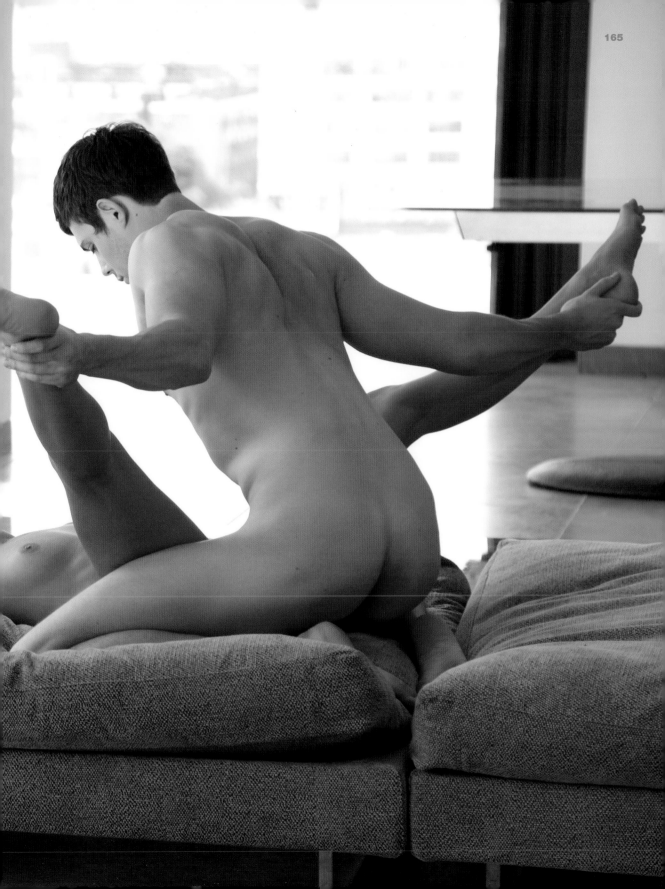

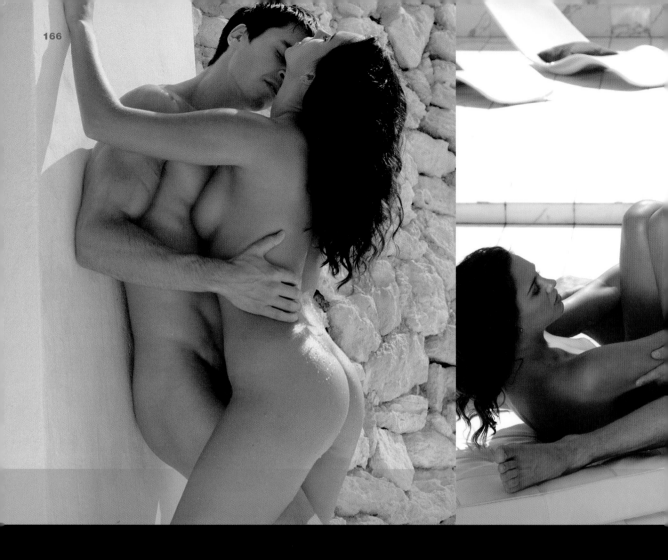

Let loose and limber up

CREATIVELY CHRISTEN EACH ROOM OF YOUR HOUSE BY TRYING THESE PROVOCATIVE POSES IN DIFFERENT ROOMS.

STAND AND DELIVER

This looks deceptively easy until you stop to think about the angle at which he's penetrating her. Some men find it uncomfortable because his penis is bent at an awkward angle and unless she keeps her bottom well and truly tilted back and upward (if that makes sense!), it tends to pop out rather frequently. So why should you try it? Because if you get it right, it's a fantastic position for one of those spur-of-the-moment screws!

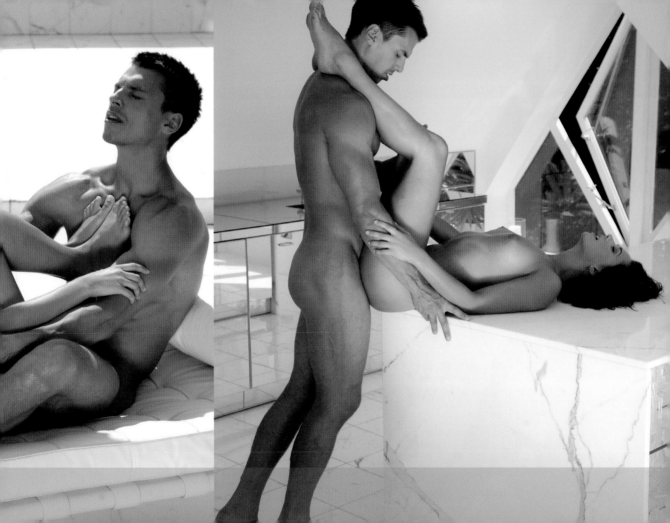

topsy-turvy

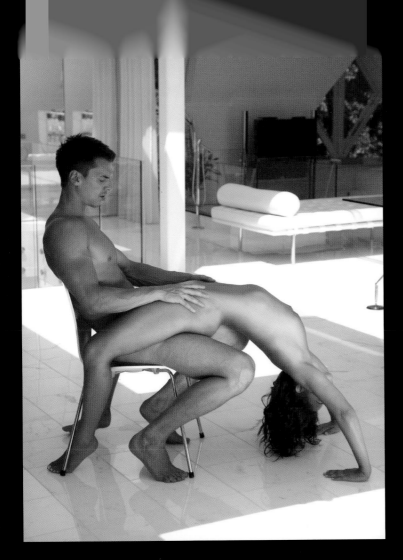

<< **STEP ONE**

Bored of watching TV on
a Sunday afternoon? This
should perk you both up
(though it's best not
attempt it with a hangover).
He perches on a chair, she
straddles his lap then, as
he hangs onto her thighs,
she leans backward in
a handstand. Taking a
moment to enjoy a rather
spectacular view of her
body, he then slides his
hands down to grip her
firmly by the waist and
prepares to stand up.

<< **STEP TWO**

You'll see this one again (like on page 178)? And you're
absolutely right—the end position is identical to the "Handstand."
It's how you got there which makes it different—and given the
Kama Sutra is all about the journey and not just the destination,
that makes sense. It's actually a simpler version (using a chair
makes it easier). You get into position more quickly, so she
needs to be completely comfortable with hanging upside down.
(He also needs to have a semi-erection because his penis is
bent down at an odd angle!). The payoffs? Yoga devotees claim
all that blood rushing to her head is good for you, both mentally
and physically. Quite why isn't explained so much.

21

TOP POSITION

the bamboo

In a beautifully choreographed lusty leg lift, she performs an erotic dance for his penis.

How to do it

She lies face up and brings her knees up to her chin. He kneels in front and penetrates, she then straightens her legs and rests them on one shoulder, pulling one leg back so it's bent. She holds onto the back of his thighs and he grips hers for balance then she "dances": alternating her leg position frequently throughout.

Why you'd want to

Her vagina is shortened so it's a tight fit for him. As she alternates the position of her legs, it alters the angle to massage his penis with a unique rolling sensation. He looks manly, and has a great view of her breasts.

Hot hint

This is already the "cheat's" version of the *Kama Sutra* "splitting of a bamboo." If you both like more challenging acrobatics, she should hook one leg on his shoulder with the other stretched out on the bed, then swap.

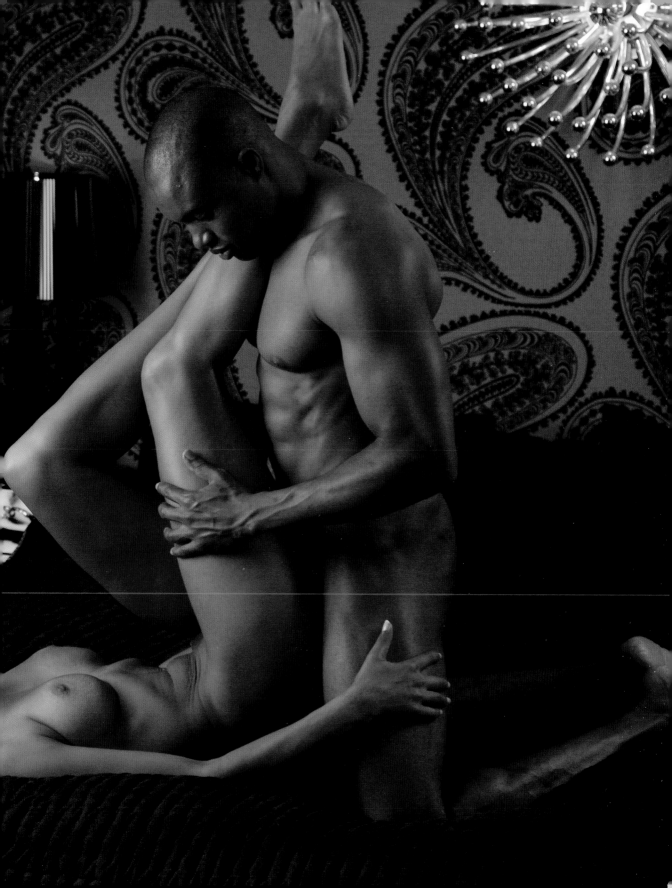

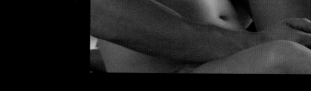

the really naughty parts

WANT TO KNOW HOW TO HAVE SEX WITH FIVE WOMEN AT ONCE, WHAT TO DO WITH ALL THE YOUNG MEN YOU'VE HIDDEN IN YOUR CLOSET, OR THE ETIQUETTE ON SHARING YOUR WIFE WITH YOUR MALE FRIENDS? THE *KAMA SUTRA* DISHES UP ALL THE DIRT!

Ancient Hindu society didn't have the same social taboos as we do today. Despite being a religious scholar, Vatsyayana doesn't just acknowledge wanting to covet your neighbor's wife, he gives detailed instructions on how to do it. Cheating isn't a sin, he had no qualms about pre-marital sex and he cheerfully instructs men on how to sneak into a harem for a guilt-free sexfest. After all, he says, the women in the harem keep each other's secrets and "a young man who enjoys all of them and who is common to them all, can continue enjoying his union with them so long as it is kept quiet." Nonjudgemental and ridiculously liberal, he obligingly describes the correct etiquette for threesomes and group sex—down to the most minute detail. There's a difference, for instance, in the way you'd conduct group sex with a courtesan (prostitute) versus sharing your own wife. He doesn't necessarily *condone* this type of behavior—there are numerous ground rules which need to be met concerning class and condition (you're only allowed to covet your neighbor's wife for instance if you're "sick with desire"). But he's not particularly concerned by it either.

The prize for "The Least Likely Sex Scenario" to happen now in real life goes to the **"Congress of a Herd of Cows"—a man satisfying five women at one time.**

There's a particularly raunchy passage where Vatsyayana talks about how women in country villages hide young men in their apartments with "highly sensual women sometimes hiding several." Greedy girlies! The young men (there's an emphasis on "young" for a reason—I doubt your average 40-year-old would be up to the task) satiate the women's desires either one by one or as a group. This scenario is for the "group." Bear in mind that biting, "beating," and scratching were all carefully controlled means of providing pleasure not pain (see page 160). Here goes:

"One holds her seated on his knees, while another takes her mouth and embraces her. One bites and scratches her, while the other penetrates her sex or licks her vulva. She is scratched, bitten, and beaten separately by one after the other, or by all together, after which they fornicate with her successively. One of the practices that satisfies a woman and calms the excitation of her hole of pleasure, the opening for the passage of liquids, or vulva, consists of one of them servicing her sex with his mouth." Well, I don't know about you but it made me wiggle a little in my seat! Vatsyayana points out that many young men enjoy a woman that may be married to one of them, either one after the other, or at the same time. How so? "One of them holds her, another enjoys her, a third uses her mouth, a fourth holds her middle part and in that way they go on enjoying her several parts alternately. The same things can be done when several men are sitting in company with one courtesan, or when one courtesan is alone with many men." (Er, aren't both those situations with the courtesan the same?) He's not sexist either: "In the same way, this can be done by the women of the King's harem when they accidentally get hold of a man." Just how you "accidentally" get hold of a man when you're in a harem, sadly, isn't explained. *Samghataka rata* is the term for having a threesome: a man making love with two women "who like each other and have the same taste" (whether this refers to clothes, men, or furniture isn't specified). "The two women lie on the same bed and the boy makes use of them both. While he is mounting one, the other, excited, kisses him and after pleasuring one he brings the other to orgasm." Threesomes also worked the other way around with two men and one woman.

The prize for "The Least Likely Sex Scenario" to happen now in real life goes to the '"Congress of a Herd of Cows"—one man satisfying five women at one time. Princes and rich merchants might well have been able to enjoy this, but for your average man today, it will probably remain a fantasy. But just in case you do find yourself surrounded by five naked, willing women, here's his advice… you lie in front of three women, giving one of them oral sex and spreading your arms to put your fingers deep inside the two other women flanking her. At the same time, you're penetrating a fourth woman who is lying underneath you with her head at the opposite end to yours. A fifth girl sits on top of the fourth girl's face, receiving cunnilingus. A cinch! Some things to think about for any couples reading this and looking at their best friends with hopeful sparkles in their eyes: group sex is different because our attitude to it has changed. Will you have added a nice, spicy fantasy to the "fantasy file," or tipped a bucket load of jealousy on your relationship? What happens if you or your partner like one of your playmates more? What happens if your partner enjoys group sex and you don't? Be warned: few couples can handle it!

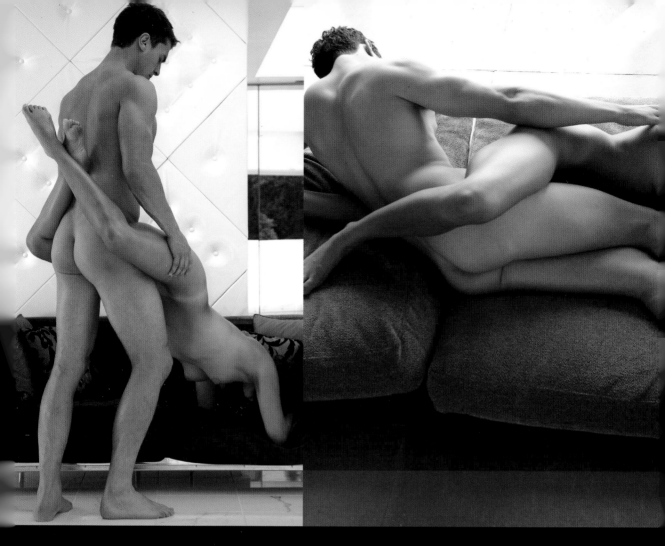

Posey positions to score points

AUDITIONING TO BE YOUR PARTNER'S MOST INVENTIVE LOVER TO DATE? JUST BRING OUT THESE BABIES AND YOU'VE GOT THE JOB!

TOMCAT

The inspiration for this comes from horny tomcats taking advantage of poor, defenseless (in heat) kitty cats. In other words, he has his wicked way and takes control. (At long last, quite frankly, after a seeming unhealthy obsession with her-on-top poses!) The difference between this and similar positions is that she clamps her legs around his back, locking her ankles. And we all know what that does, don't we! Yes, a tighter vaginal canal—and that means better sex for everyone!

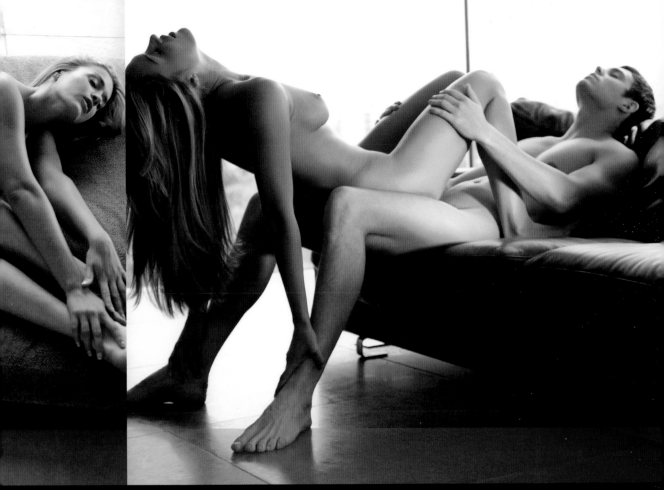

TOP-TO-TOE

This looks damn impressive but the truth is, if you've had side-by-side sex, you've probably done a similar version without even realizing it. Just no one took a picture of you at the time (or at least you hope they didn't). The only difference is, instead of facing the same way, you're lying in opposite directions (head pointed toward each other's feet). Thing is, most women move down the bed to make penetration easier and this simply exaggerates that natural movement. It's easy, it's fun, it's familiar. Go for it!

EDGY

It looks precarious—and it is. The trick to her not falling to the floor is him keeping his thighs firmly in place, positioned underneath her hips. Get too overexcited, let them fall apart and you have… well, let's hope an unhappy girlfriend is all you have to cope with! He slouches back on the couch, she sits on his lap, then carefully leans backward, hands on his calves and feet on the sofa by his side. In that position, you're both supposed to meditate about life, love, lust… how cool your new ceiling light is.

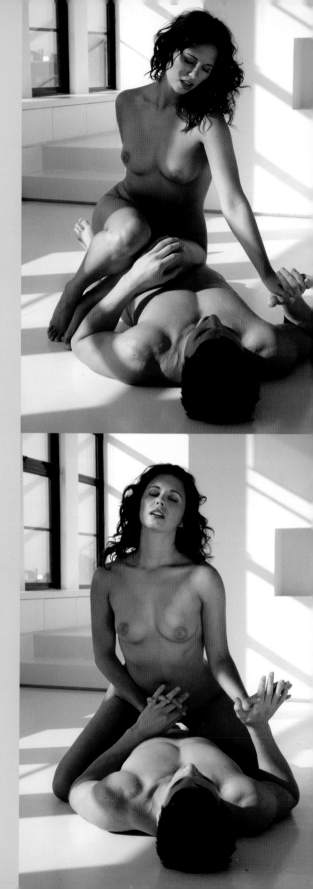

22

TOP POSITION

spinning top

This involves her sitting on his penis, then swiveling around on it like a spinning top. Yes, it is a totally crazy idea!

How to do it

Even Vatsyayana strongly urges you to practice this a lot (like, no kidding!), but if you break it down into stages it can work in a wobbly type of way! She starts by assuming the usual her-on-top position (see right, bottom) then (very slowly and carefully) lifts one leg over his body (see right, top) so both her legs are on one side. The next move is to turn her body so she's now facing away from him (see opposite, main image).

Why you'd want to

Some sexperts would strongly suggest you *don't* try this one, proclaiming it downright dangerous! I agree—by attempting the swivel as *one movement* is about as sensible as putting his penis in a blender, turning it on and seeing what happens. Doing it in stages, though, can be a fun challenge. Just be careful for God's sake!

Hot hint

She should squeeze those pelvic floor muscles tight to stop him from falling out!

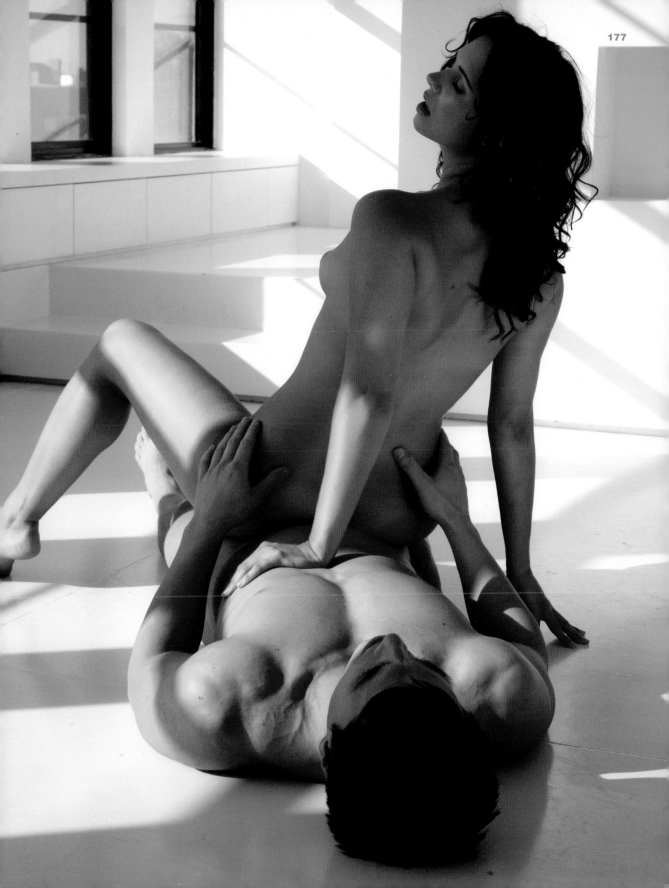

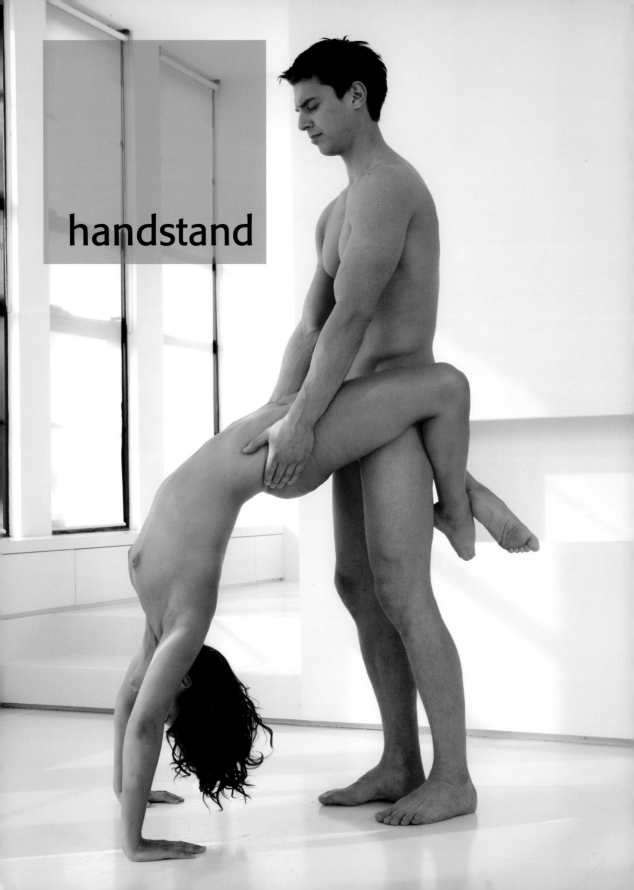

handstand

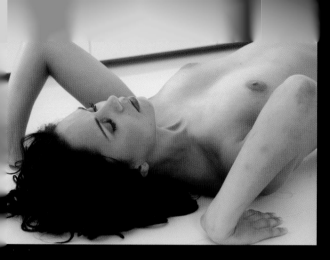

<< STEP ONE

Now we're talking! This is one of those positions that makes us all go "Yikes!" and feel envious of those athletic bastards who are so fit and flexible, the handstand is their equivalent of our missionary. Take it from me, it isn't. But even if you end up in a heap on the floor, it's worth a laugh. Start with her flat on the floor, her bottom raised and feet in line with her hips. She then brings her hands up by her ears, turning them so her fingertips point downward.

>> STEP TWO

She arches her back, lifting her hips in the air and dropping her head back. He supports her as she arches, kneeling on one leg and holding her upper thighs and/or hips. This part is actually harder than the final step, so hang in there. Literally.

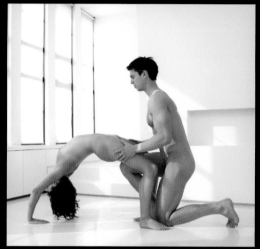

STEP THREE

He stands up s-l-o-w-l-y, still holding on tight to her, moving his hands to support her lower back. She's now completely upside down, but while it looks like she's supporting her own weight, he's taking most of the strain and her hands are on the ground

V for stability.
V

<< STEP FOUR

He completely straightens up and she crosses her feet behind his back. The payoff? It's perfect positioning to hit her G-spot. Because it's impossible for her to do much other than, well, stand there upside down, it's up to him to move her back and forth. Whether you've both got the stamina to actually reach climax in the handstand remains to be seen.

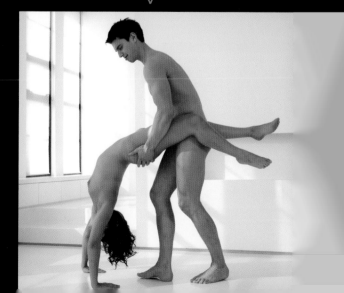

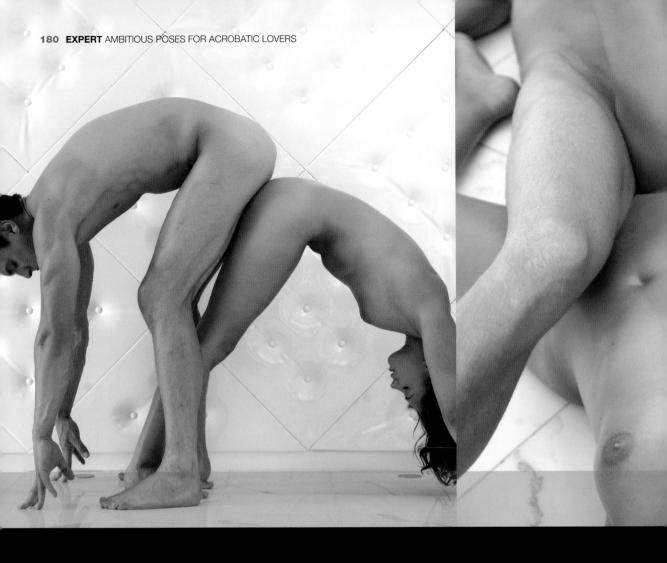

Ambitious poses for acrobatic lovers

AND I'M NOT KIDDING WHEN I SAY AMBITIOUS. THE "BOTTOMS UP" ONE RATES HIGH ON THE OH-MY-GOD FACTOR, BUT THE OTHER TWO ARE ACHIEVABLE. IF NOTHING ELSE, YOU'LL HAVE A GOOD LAUGH TRYING!

BOTTOMS UP

Yes, I am putting you on. Unless he has a long or curved penis, you can practice this one all you like, but it just ain't going to happen! It's officially called "autumn dog" and it comes to you courtesy of Tao. Not that you'll be coming by doing it, mind you. It's inspired by the mating of dogs, hence the charming name. Both of you bend over so your bottoms are touching, her raised on tiptoes to allow him to penetrate. Yeah right.

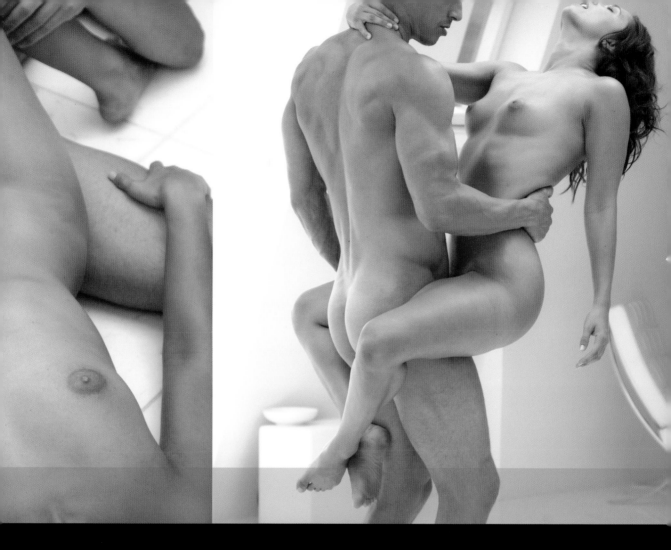

CRISSCROSS

This is actually designed as a post-sex position: a relaxing way to stay sexually connected while you're both basking in the afterglow of an orgasm. I think it's actually a great way to get you there! Scissoring your legs, slide in to meet each other, using your hands to bend his penis to penetrate. You can hang onto whatever body part you like to give yourselves leverage to thrust. Grab each other's wrist if you're having problems

COCKY TARZAN

The difference between this and Tarzan (see page 129), is that the women leans back as far as possible, so her torso is virtually at right angles to his. How come it doesn't look like that in the photo? Err… because it's damn hard to do, that's why! You need long arms, a brave constitution, and strong thigh muscles to grip his. Personally, I'd give myself a gold star for accomplishing Tarzan and give this one a pass.

23

TOP POSITION

lotus

The infamous yoga position just got one hell of a lot more interesting. Forget "omm," this is all about "ahhhhhh."

How to do it

A sexy staple for spiritual devotees, this is classic *Kama Sutra* so well worth trying. "Trying" being the operative word. It's quite easy to get into position but so uncomfortable staying in it, you're more likely to grit your teeth than grunt with orgasmic bliss. She lies back, crosses her legs and draws them up to her chest. He kneels, his legs flanking her hips, and penetrates.

Why you'd want to

The purpose behind it is sort of sexy: it's designed to draw the vagina up to meet the penis. But unless you're top of your yoga class (show off!) it doesn't really do what it says on the box i.e. penis and vagina are waving at each other, but that's about it. Why attempt it? So that you can say you've at least given *Kama Sutra* sex a try!

Hot hint

If you want to try the *true* lotus position, she should try tucking her heels into her hip sockets, rather than simply crossing her legs. Err, good luck!!

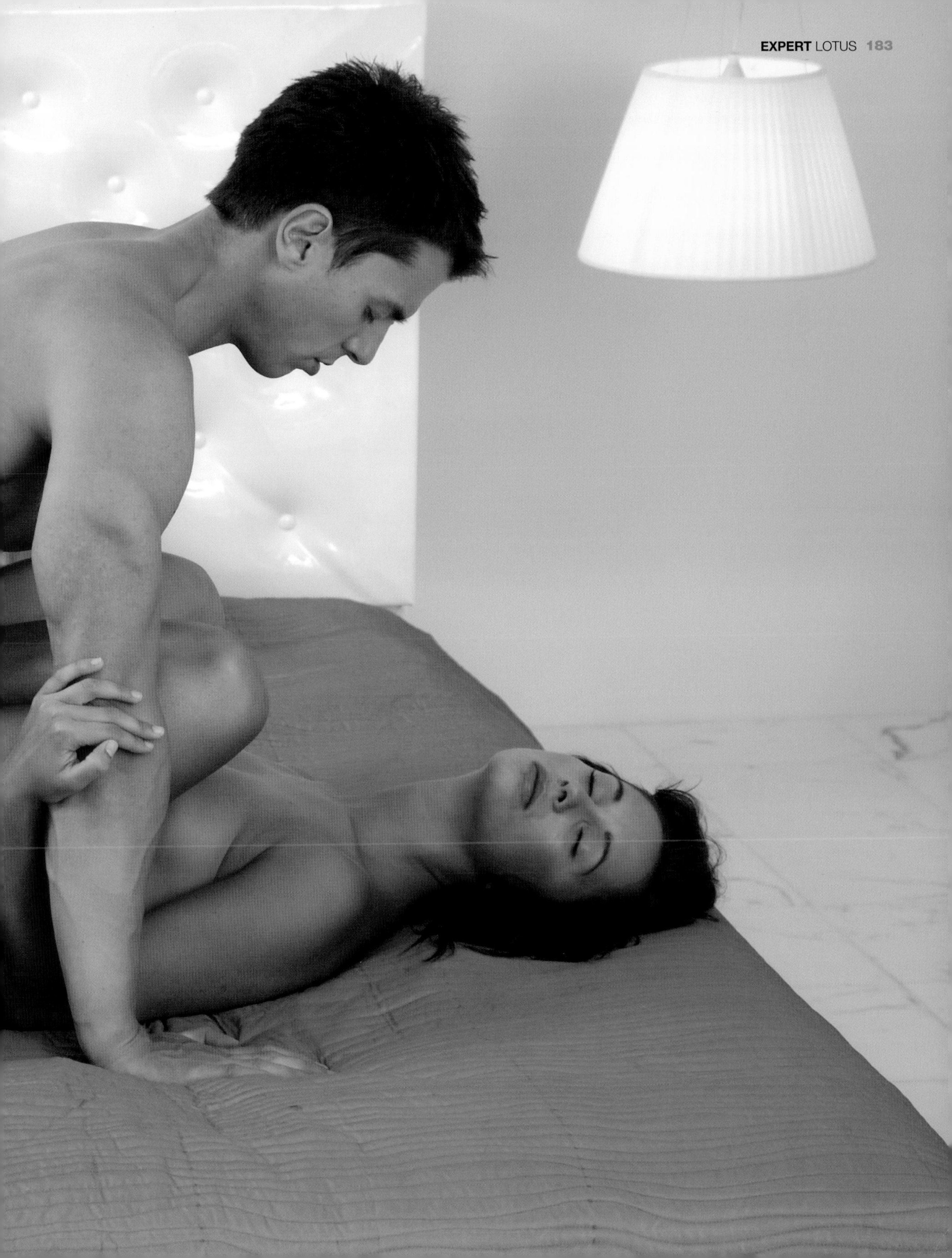

hang ten

<< STEP ONE

He kneels at her feet, worshipping her as the goddess she is (OK, I just made that bit up, but he does need to kneel). She sits on his lap and you both get as close as possible, him relishing the feel of her breasts squashed between you and both luxuriating in the feel of skin on skin.

STEP TWO

She pulls back and raises herself slightly to allow him to penetrate. Again, it's not cheating to use your hands to guide him in! Revert back to the same position you adopted in step one, except this time he is inside. No thrusting at this point, instead she contracts and releases her pelvic floor muscles.

V
V

<< STEP THREE

He stands as she holds on tight, keeping his knees bent. He then carefully lowers her so she's sitting as low as possible while still maintaining penetration. It's hard to do much more than simply bash against each other, so keep the pelvic floor "milking" motion going. If you like finishing with some good old-fashioned vigorous thrusting, it's relatively easy for him to plonk her down on an appropriate height piece of furniture.

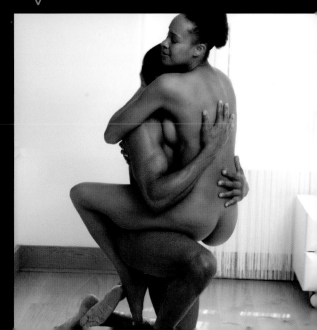

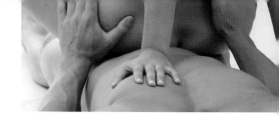

the crazy bits

DEVIOUS WAYS TO MAKE YOUR PENIS GROW, HOW TO BREAK INTO A HAREM, THE GIRLS YOU SHOULD MARRY—AND THOSE YOU CAN SCREW GUILT-FREE. THE GLORIOUSLY POLITICALLY INCORRECT TAKE ON HOW TO RUN YOUR LIFE, ACCORDING TO THE *KAMA SUTRA*!

OK, this isn't strictly about sex but anyone who reads the *Kama Sutra* can't help but let out the odd stunned guffaw at a lot of the advice. Yes, it probably all made sense 2,000 years ago, but today it's either so politically incorrect or downright unbelievable, it's hilarious. I couldn't resist sharing. This is a mere taste of the funny bits.

To increase his libido, he should **drink sugared milk in which he has boiled up a goat's testicle.**. Come on, they must be for sale somewhere…

Get him back… by turning yourself into a cow

So here's the deal: you're a deserted wife, so you cast a spell to get your husband back. Instead of using today's tactics (lose truck loads of weight, buy a killer black dress, and be seen out with a boy toy), you instead pray to a sacred cow causing hubby to have a dream of a cow with your face superimposed on it. Instead of seeing the irony ("She really was a cow!"), he sees your beauty "anew." Rushing home, he embraces you so ardently you almost suffocate. But this is a good thing. You're both so turned on, you have make-up sex—aptly titled (given the cow connection) "churning the milk"—which involves him "turning his penis around inside your delicious vagina."

And, if you're choosing a wife, check that she's got no "hidden" faults—a hook nose, upturned nostrils, male genitalia (!) or crooked thighs. And if you're looking for a woman with real standing, you'd be well advised to avoid taking a wife and instead opt for a courtesan (fancy prostitute). Courtesans were the only women who enjoyed financial and social independence and were acknowledged as being clever, witty, interesting, and talented. Equals of the powerful men who sought them out.

HOW TO BREAK INTO A HAREM

According to Vatsyayana, it's easier to screw one of the king's wives than your sexy neighbor. Apparently, nowhere is as poorly guarded as a harem—and no women more accessible than the wives of the king. An "enterprising" (aka desperately horny) young man can choose from a variety of ways to get inside. First option: hide yourself in a barrel and wait for a servant to carry it inside. (Boring—been done too many times in films.) Or masquerade yourself as a maid. Despite having muscles, a moustache (popular back then), hands the size of dinner plates, and an enormous Adam's apple, the lazy sentries and overworked servants aren't going to notice, says Vatsyayana. The last way is my favorite: take a potion that will make you invisible, but the outcome is "uncertain" (like, even he didn't believe it). The ingredients? Burn the eyes of a serpent and smear a paste of the ashes on your eyelids. Why is the vision of a two-year-old covering their eyes and saying, "You can't see me" dancing before *my* eyes.

… and how to sneak a man into a harem

Because women in a harem have to share one man, sexual frustration is high. They're as eager to smuggle men in, as men are eager to get in there! So how did they manage? Well, some dressed up as men and used the bulbous root as a dildo. As you do. Others "worked themselves into a frenzy" on the phallus of a statue. More obvious (and pleasurable): persuading one of the eunuch guards to give them oral sex—or indulging in a good old lesbian romp with each other.

But "the best and most dangerous" sexual treat was to smuggle a man into the royal apartments. As before, he could use the magic potion to make himself invisible (and get instantly arrested because it doesn't work) or disguise himself as a woman. Another innovative idea: arrive rolled in a carpet! (Who actually takes the carpet inside isn't clear). Shrewdly, Vatsyayana hints that a good time to smuggle him in is during "the confused comings and goings that surround a drinking festival" (everyone's so sloshed, they can't focus). Clever man.

MAKE A MAGIC POTION

Using common ingredients everyone has in their kitchen cupboard (not), these concoctions were suggested to cure the following:

• **To enlarge a penis** Rub it with the bristles of certain insects, then for 10 nights rub it with oil, followed by another treatment of the bristly insects. After this, (not surprisingly) your "lingam" will be so swollen you'll have to lie down and let it hang through a hole in the bed (What? Your bed doesn't have a handy hole in it?). You then massage it with cooling ointments. After the pain disappears (and if you still want some after all this rigmarole), you'll find the swelling remains. Now, if only you could find the girl you'd planned to bed all those weeks before…

• **To turn an ugly person into a magnetic beauty** You know the story, they're either ugly and interesting or gorgeous and dull. Happily, here's a simple solution: secretly get them to eat the pollen of the blue lotus with ghee and honey or tie a gilded peacock or hyena to their right hand. There! Problem solved.

PICK THE RIGHT GIRL

Vatsyayana offers up copious lists detailing which women are suitable for what. This is but a sample…

• **Enjoy guilt-free:** virgins, women who've been married twice, courtesans or public women (poor servant types). Enjoyed it? Well, you're only allowed to get attached to the first one and—surprise, surprise!—it's the virgin! She's the only one suitable for marrying and bearing children.

• **Don't go near**—lepers, lunatics, women who tell secrets, women who ask for sex in public, women who are too pale and white, or too dark and black, women who smell bad—or female friends.

• **For a one-night stand**—women who spend a lot of time chatting to neighbors, who look sideways at you, childless women, an actor's wife, poor women, the wife of a man who has many younger brothers, vain women, women whose husbands travel, jealous women, lazy women, a humpback, a dwarf, and loud and vulgar women.

reading list

If you're interested in finding out more about spiritual sex, I'd highly recommend any of these books.

The Art of Sexual Magic
(Piatkus, 1995)
By Margo Anand
Highly acclaimed and informative (for true disciples!)

The Multi-Orgasmic Woman
(Rodale, 2005)
By Mantak Chia and Dr. Rachel Carlton Abrams
The ultimate handbook for achieving multi-orgasm for her

The Multi-Orgasmic Man
(Thorsons, 2001)
By Mantak Chia and Douglas Abrams Arava
Fantastic guide to multiple orgasm for him

Deepak Chopra Kama Sutra
(Virgin Books, 2006)
By Deepak Chopra
Elegant and articulate take on spiritual sex

The Cosmo Kama Sutra
(Hearst Communications, 2004)
By the Editors of Cosmopolitan
Fun positions book

Teach Yourself Tantric Sex
(Teach Yourself, 2003)
By Richard Craze
Good, easy to understand overview

The Complete Kama Sutra
(Park Street Press, 1994)
Translated by Alain Danielou
Excellent, accurate translation of the original

Kama Sutra for 21st-Century Lovers
(Dorling Kindersley, 2003)
By Anne Hooper
Great all-rounder

The Women's Kama Sutra
(Vega, 2001)
By Nitya Lacroix
A female take on spiritual sex

Tantra Between the Sheets
(Amorata Press, 2003)
By Val Sampson
Great, user-friendly guide to Tantric sex

The Modern Kama Sutra
(HarperElement, 2005)
By Kamini and Kirk Thomas
Good overview

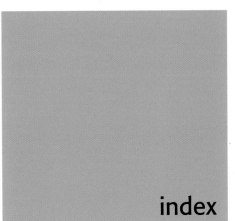

index

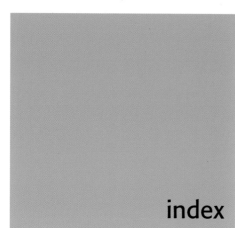

index

acknowledgments

This is my seventh book about sex, and my 11th book in total and I'm extremely happy to say, I have had the pleasure of working with pretty much the same people for each one. I've thanked you all profusely in the past, but just in case you haven't got the message of how much I treasure you all…

To my family, Shirley, Terry, Patrick, Maureen, Nigel, Diana, Deborah, Doug, Charlie, and Maddy. They say families aren't perfect but by God, you come close!

To my agent and best friend, Vicki McIvor. Humblest thanks, as always, for being such a support in my life in all ways possible. I am so lucky to have you!

To all my closest, dearest friends, Sandra Aldridge, Peggy Bunker, Rachel Corcoran, Claire Faragher, Catherine Jarvie, and Fenella Thomas. Thanks for being so patient with me, even though we all know I'm a workaholic, and for making me laugh even when stress levels were at their highest.

To Richard Stay, my deliciously quirky, funny, patient, sexy, and loving boyfriend. I am so enjoying having you in my life!

To the couples who road-tested positions. I know you don't want to be named but surely it's obvious who you are by the various, unexplained injuries?

To my editor, Dawn Bates, for not only doing a superb job (as usual), but for laughing at all my jokes (even those you rather swiftly edited out).

To Peter Jones at DK, who's been there with me from the start and never once failed to be anything but outstandingly supportive and ridiculously patient. Thanks for always humoring me.

To my book designers, Nigel Wright and Bev Speight at XAB, for turning my words into such a visual treat.

To Stephanie Jackson at DK, for being such an enthusiastic fan of my work and inspiration for me to come up with even more funky, fresh new titles.

And to all at Dorling Kindersley, world-wide, enormous thanks for everything. In the UK office, John Roberts, Deborah Wright, Serena Stent, Hermoine Ireland, Liz Statham, Catherine Bell, Adèle Hayward, Helen Spencer, and Katherine Raj. In the US office, Gary June, Therese Burke, Tom Korman, and Rachel Kempster, and in Canada, Chris Houston and Loraine Taylor.

Spirit and flesh have never been separate.
They keep apart just to flirt.